The Complete Book
of Home Exercise

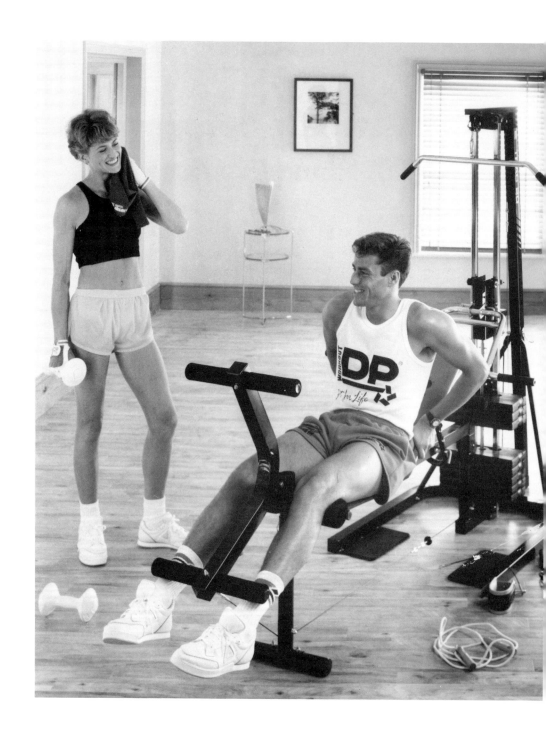

The Complete Book of
HOME EXERCISE

TONY LYCHOLAT

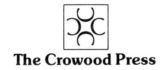

The Crowood Press

First published in 1990 by
The Crowood Press
Ramsbury, Marlborough,
Wiltshire SN8 2HE

British Library Cataloguing in Publication Data

Lycholat, Tony
  The Complete Book of Home Exercise.
  1. Physical fitness. Exercises
  I. Title
  613.7'1

ISBN 1 85223 333 8

Typeset by Action Typesetting Limited, Gloucester
Printed in Great Britain at The Bath Press

Contents

Acknowledgements

As with the companion title in this series, *The Complete Book of Diet and Exercise*, thanks to everyone who helped in the writing and production of this book. Special thanks must go to Reebok who were kind enough to provide clothing and footwear, as well as photographs of Tim Hutchings. Roy Wooding did a great job, behind the camera, as did Kate Gowar, who spent much of her time in front of it. Thanks.

1 The Benefits of Exercise

Regular exercise is rapidly becoming accepted as an essential aspect of everyone's life. Few people – if any – do no physical activity at all. To give just a few examples, it has been estimated that as many as nine million adults in the British Isles walk for fitness and recreational benefits; around four million people go to keep fit and aerobics classes on a regular basis; some two million individuals go jogging; approximately five million people go swimming and over one million people can be found cycling for fitness. Participation in all of these sports and activities, as well as in many not mentioned, has also seen quite dramatic increases in the last few years, both in this country and abroad.

Many reasons have been given for the public's massive interest in physical activity and fitness in general. Certainly it is true that the facilities for leisure and recreation have improved dramatically over the last ten years. This, coupled with increased leisure time, and harnessed to fitness campaigns promoted by bodies like the Sports Council in Great Britain and similar authorities in other countries, has certainly made the general public more aware of what is on offer from the point of view of leisure and recreation. Yet the most important stimulus for getting people to exercise on a regular basis has been that generated by research indicating the link between physical fitness, health, well-being and general appearance.

Early links between physical activity and health were first illustrated in the 1960s by Dr Kenneth Cooper in America, (although to be fair, the Ancient Greeks had pointed out that for a body to be healthy, it needed regular physical activity). Cooper's work was influential, though, precisely because it simply indicated the link between physical inactivity and a high risk of heart disease – America's number one killer. Based upon his research, Cooper formulated a simple series of physical assessment tests and activity programmes, concentrated around aerobic exercise (walking, jogging, cycling, swimming) which could be followed by anyone. Cooper's activity programmes took off in a big way, and the people of America found themselves with a new word – aerobics – in their vocabulary. With a great deal of inflammatory media hype, aerobics took off, although to be honest, early regular exercisers tended to be men who took up jogging and running. It wasn't until aerobic exercise was modified to incorporate dance steps by Jackie Sorensen in the 1970s that women began exercising in a big way. Aerobic dance had been born and soon a whole nation, men and women were regularly doing some form of aerobic activity. Naturally enough, other countries followed suit, with the aerobics boom hitting a peak in Great Britain around 1981 – 2.

Since then, interest has not declined, despite the comments of many inactive journalists. Instead, the fitness industry has grown steadily. Aerobic exercise in all forms is as popular as ever, and other forms of exercise for other components of fitness (weight training for strength, stretching for flexibility, for example) are becoming increasingly popular. People are mixing and matching their exercise activities ('cross-training') to achieve a balanced approach to fitness, and finding that regular appropriate exercise can achieve tremendous results both in terms of the way they look and the way they feel. And as more and more research is completed, more and more positive links between fitness, health and well-being are being firmly established. Fitness is now neither fad nor fashion, it is socially acceptable, great fun and essential for survival: and science can prove it.

Once exercise became more popular, as often happens in science, more and more researchers began to investigate its reported benefits. The mass of data that has now been accumulated makes for interesting reading, and puts the case for regular exercise more strongly than ever before. The most researched area has been aerobic exercise, as you might imagine. Aerobic exercise is basically any activity which uses large muscle groups in rhythmical contractions which can be continued for at least ten minutes. Into this category come many activities such as those already mentioned: walking, jogging, swimming, cycling and aerobic dance. Research has indicated that it is this type of exercise, carried out for long enough, often enough, which is most effective when it comes to reducing your risk of heart disease and circulatory problems. Aerobic exercise may also lower blood pressure, decrease the levels of harmful circulating fats in your bloodstream and help in the prevention and treatment of obesity and adult-onset diabetes.

Of great interest recently has also been the role of regular aerobic exercise in the prevention of the condition known as osteoporosis. Basically, osteoporosis is a condition in which the bones of the skeleton become increasingly fragile as they lose bone mass and density. It affects women more than men, is part and parcel of the ageing process, and is now recognised as a major public health problem worldwide. Generally speaking, as many as 30 per cent of all women may find themselves suffering from osteoporosis to a greater or lesser extent, especially following the menopause, with white women of small bone mass who are relatively inactive and who have dietary deficiencies being particularly vulnerable. Research has indicated that regular weight-bearing aerobic exercise can be extremely useful in retarding bone loss. It would seem that the stress exerted upon bone by the exercise in question makes the bone stronger and denser and less liable to fractures. Incidentally, those same stresses which make bones stronger also seem to make the joints stronger at the same time, making them less susceptible to injury.

Yet besides such relatively obvious functional, physical changes, research over the last few years has also focused upon psychological changes associated with regular aerobic exercise. Most regular exercisers have long argued that their exercise programme leaves them feeling less stressed and more relaxed. Psychological studies have now reinforced these anecdotal reports. Not only can aerobic exercise cause the release of hormones which can promote a sense of well-being, it can also lead to a general improvement in a person's feeling of self-worth and hence self-image. Such positive effects associated with an aerobic exercise programme have led to the use of exercise in the treatment of depression and other similar psychological disorders. And, on a less clinical level, many companies have now realised that the provision of exercise facilities can help workers get rid of pent-up aggression related to their occupations, as well as making them fitter, more able employees.

Aerobic exercise obviously has a lot going for it, but as important as it is, other aspects of fitness also have to be considered, since they also offer quite dramatic health benefits. Generally speaking, physical fitness can be broken down into a number of component parts. These may be divided into two subgroups: those components of fitness which are most important with respect to health (health-

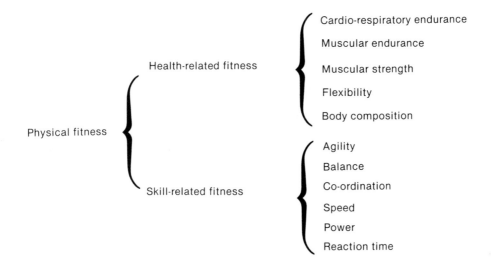

Physical fitness
- Health-related fitness
  - Cardio-respiratory endurance
  - Muscular endurance
  - Muscular strength
  - Flexibility
  - Body composition
- Skill-related fitness
  - Agility
  - Balance
  - Co-ordination
  - Speed
  - Power
  - Reaction time

Fig 1   Components of physical fitness.

related components); and those components of fitness which are most important with respect to the execution of certain skills (skill-related components). This breakdown of components of physical fitness is indicated in *Fig 1*, and each component is further discussed in the relevant chapter.

Briefly, different types of exercise improve or enhance different components of fitness. Aerobic exercise does little for muscular strength, for example, yet possessing muscular strength is very important in terms of your health, since it allows you to lift, carry and move objects — as well as yourself — with relative ease. Similarly, running may be great aerobic exercise for the body in general and will also improve the endurance of the muscles of the lower body: but it won't do much for the endurance of the muscles of the upper body. It is appropriate muscular endurance, coupled with the right blend of strength and flexibility, which is so important if you are to have good posture and avoid posture-related ailments, including a large number of back problems.

Flexibility exercises also keep the joints supple and mobile as well as enabling you to reach, bend, twist and turn with ease. In other words, if you are to get all the researched health and fitness benefits of regular exercise, one type of exercise is not enough. As more and more people are coming to realise, total fitness is the key.

Yet as persuasive as the health benefits of regular exercise are, a survey in a fitness magazine in Britain indicated that most people exercise on a regular basis in order to bring about changes in their appearance, and not for health reasons. Yet as with health benefits, the best way to achieve positive changes in appearance through exercise is through a combination of exercise activities. Aerobic exercise, for example, if it is of long duration (20 minutes plus) and low intensity and repeated regularly is the type of exercise which is most effective in using up body fat as fuel. In combination with an appropriate diet, aerobic exercise is the most effective way of getting rid of excess fat. However, if you want to tone up all your muscles, some form of strength and muscular endurance programme, linked with appropriate mobility work is the answer. Obviously, if you want all the possible shaping benefits of exercise, cross-training is the best way. Mixing and matching exercise activities in this way also allows you to emphasise different fitness, health and shape benefits, as well as allowing you − if you so wish − to work on specific parts of the body. In fact, within the limitations of your own genetics, dedication and time, there is very little you cannot achieve with the right blend of exercise activities and an appropriate exercise programme.

Another very important point to realise is that exercise is not just the province of the young fit-looking adult, who is invariably depicted 'working-out' in magazines and on television. (In fact, the worse condition you are in, the more dramatic your improvement!) Exercise can produce positive health, fitness and shape benefits regardless of your age and initial fitness level. To illustrate this point it is worth considering some facts with regard to exercise and older age groups (fifty years' old plus).

It is largely acknowledged that between the ages of thirty and seventy, the body begins to undergo a process which is generally referred to as 'functional decline'. Some of the physiological changes which accompany this process include an average decrease in work capacity of around 30 per cent; a decrease in muscle mass of between 25 and 30 per cent; a decrease in flexibility of up to 30 per cent, and an increase in blood pressure. Nerve conduction velocities also fall, bone loss (as has been indicated) is quite marked, and there are also quite dramatic decreases in lung and kidney function. Resting metabolic rate also falls by around 10 per cent. Yet whilst much of the functional decline associated with getting older is due to the ageing process itself and is irreversible, there is a considerable amount of evidence to support the view that many of the decreases in physiological function are due to disuse. Indeed, some authorities have argued that up to 50 per cent of the functional decline noted in older, otherwise healthy individuals is due to inactivity. Effectively, what this means is that whilst we cannot reverse the ageing process itself and the functional decline which accompanies it, regular appropriate physical activity should enable us to slow this process down. As evidence of this, at the Institute for Aerobics Research in Dallas, researchers have assessed the fitness levels of many thousands of people of all ages and have found many instances of men of retirement age who, having maintained a high level of physical activity all their lives, can easily out-perform inactive, sedentary men in their twenties when it comes to tests of physical fitness. Once again, the Ancient Greeks first observed this phenomenon, with Hippocrates noting that unused and idle bodies become liable to disease, are often defective in growth and age quickly.

Fortunately, more and more older adults are taking up exercise, especially in Great Britain, with activity programmes for the fifty-plus age group being promoted heavily by the Sports Council. Fortunately, too, the old wives' tales surrounding exercise and older people are rapidly being dismissed. Older individuals are responsive to training, although admittedly the rate of improvement is often not as marked as in younger people. And it is becoming increasingly obvious that it really is never too late to start, whatever your reasons for exercising. This fact is certainly backed up by scientific research looking at the effects of exercise programmes on people as old as eighty-eight, who have responded dramatically with improvements in all parameters measured.

However, the young should not be complacent and sit idly until they are thirty years old. It has been observed that many problems which manifest themselves later in adult life (heart disease, for example), may begin in childhood as a result of lack of physical activity and poor diet. The old saying that 'a fat child becomes a fat adult' is also largely true, and obesity is a major cause of illness in Western societies. Exercise and dietary habits do need to be established in childhood and adolescence if they are to become part of an individual's lifestyle. Many of today's children are actually far more inactive than their parents were as children. Shocking statistics show that it is not uncommon for many children to spend as much as five hours a day immobile in front of a television screen. The change in the physical education structure in Britain also means that many children are actually doing less formal exercise and sport than ever before. In the light of such information, children and adolescents will certainly profit from being introduced to the principles of exercise outlined in this text. Younger people are also in the fortunate position of being able to exercise as the body is growing. An appropriate exercise programme at this time means that the training effect — exercise results and benefits — are that much greater. In view of this, that old saying should perhaps be revised to read: 'a fit, active child becomes a fit, active adult'.

Whichever way you look at it, exercise offers all kinds of benefits to all kinds of people. Obviously certain rules have to be followed if everybody is to get the most from their exercise programme, and some of these rules are slightly different according to your age, fitness level and reasons for exercising. Naturally enough, all the information you will need to exercise effectively is included in this book in the appropriate section.

Hopefully, having read this far, you will now be convinced that exercise is of great benefit to you. The only thing that could possibly dissuade you from the next step —

actually exercising — is the potential inaccessibility of your chosen exercise activities. You may think that exercise has to be done in a gym, exercise studio or sports centre. Whilst certain activities do require specialist equipment and facilities, many do not. In fact many activities can be done either in your own home, or around the streets and parks surrounding your home. It is quite possible to design an exercise programme which is fully comprehensive in terms of fitness and which requires no equipment whatsoever, other than exercise clothing and footwear. The purchase of simple equipment which can be used at home (weights, cycle, etc.) naturally increases the total number of exercise options open to you, but may not be necessary in your case, since what you need reflects your fitness requirements and exercise preferences.

There are other advantages to exercising at home, too. Certainly you'll always be able to exercise whenever you want to. For the busy person, this is often the only way they will be able to incorporate a fitness programme into their normal lifestyle. Home exercising is also private, and for many people this is essential. Not everyone likes to exercise in the company of others, for whatever reason. Home exercise can also be a social time for families and is a great way of introducing the concept of fitness and regular exercise to children. Having fitness facilities at home can also save you time, particularly if you are used to travelling to a gym or sports centre to do something which could quite easily be done at home: you'll certainly save travelling and parking time. By now it should be quite clear that there are obvious advantages to working out at home. Naturally, exercising at home needs a little forethought, especially if you are intending to purchase various items of exercise equipment, but that's what this book is all about. At the end of this book you should know exactly what you need both in terms of fitness and equipment, how much room any item of equipment needs, how much it will cost, how to choose the best, and how to put together an exercise programme that works, whatever your goal. Finally, you'll be able to achieve all your fitness aims from the comfort and privacy of your own home.

2 How Fit are You?

This chapter is all about assessing yourself. Essentially the information given here will enable you to work out with reasonable accuracy just how fit you are at the moment. This is essential for several reasons. Firstly, a fitness assessment lets you know exactly where you are starting from. This means that when it comes to planning your exercise programme, you will be starting from the right place. Secondly, a fitness assessment gives you some idea of how fit you are in relationship to a general population. Thirdly, regular fitness assessments allow you to measure and monitor the effectiveness of your exercise programme. Finally, a fitness assessment will also allow you to work out your fitness requirements.

The first step in any fitness assessment involves answering a few simple questions. Whilst it is true that everyone can benefit from an exercise programme, those individuals who have been relatively inactive for a number of years, or who are unsure of their current health status should complete what is commonly called a 'Pre-exercise question-naire'. *Fig 2* is a typical questionnaire. Answer the questions listed as truthfully as possible. You should consult your GP if you can answer

---

These questions are designed to assess your suitability for exercise. Please answer each question as accurately as possible, reading each question carefully.

	YES	NO
1. Have your ever suffered from heart disease, high blood pressure or any other cardio-vascular problem?	☐	☐
2. Is there any history of heart disease in your family?	☐	☐
3. Have you ever been troubled by accountable or unaccountable chest pain, or tightness in the chest, especially if associated with minimal effort?	☐	☐
4. Are you prone to headaches, fainting or dizziness?	☐	☐
5. Have you any medical condition which you think might interfere with your participation in an exercise programme?	☐	☐
6. Do you suffer from pain or limited movement in any joint?	☐	☐
7. Are you taking any drugs or medication at the moment, or recovering from a recent illness or operation?	☐	☐
8. Are you extremely overweight, or extremely underweight?	☐	☐
9. Are you pregnant?	☐	☐
10. Are you a newcomer to exercise and aged over 35?	☐	☐

Fig 2   Pre-exercise questionnaire

'yes' to any of the ten questions. Positive answers do not mean that you should not exercise, merely that you may need to adapt your exercise programme in some manner. Your GP will advise you accordingly. If you answer 'no' to all of the questions, yet have some misgivings about your general state of health, do not hesitate in obtaining specialist advice before starting an exercise programme.

Assuming you are fit to exercise, the next stage of the assessment procedure is to work out just how fit you are. Because physical fitness comprises many different components (see *Fig 1*), a number of different tests must be completed if you are to obtain an overall picture of your total fitness. Generally speaking, the most important components of fitness for recreational exercisers (as opposed to competitive sports performers) are the health-related components. Assessing the skill-related components is of less general interest and tests of these components do not fall within the scope of this text.

ASSESSING CARDIO-RESPIRATORY ENDURANCE

Technically, cardio-respiratory endurance is an expression of how effectively you can get oxygen into the body, deliver it to the working muscles and use it to provide energy, whilst at the same time removing any waste products from the muscles which may limit continuous physical activity. Generally speaking, a person with a high level of cardio-respiratory endurance may be assumed to be 'aerobically fit'. The benefits of aerobic fitness have been listed in detail in the previous chapter and the reader should be in no doubt as to the considerable advantages of having a high degree of aerobic fitness.

Essentially, the measurement of someone's cardio-respiratory endurance is useful since it reflects their aerobic fitness and gives a very useful indication of the functional capacity of their oxygen transporting capacity. Assessing cardio-respiratory endurance/aerobic fitness can be done in several ways. In the clinical confines of the laboratory, exercise physiologists will attempt to measure an individual's maximal oxygen uptake, which is the greatest volume of oxygen which can be used by the cells of the body per unit of time. This is the 'true' measure of cardio-respiratory efficiency. Such a test usually requires exercise to exhaustion on a cycle or treadmill, with expired air collections being made throughout the test. The air collected is then analysed and the individual's maximal oxygen uptake is computed. Such an assessment requires extremely expensive equipment and highly trained personnel to perform the test.

Far simpler, though less accurate tests can be carried out with the minimum of equipment. One of the simplest tests, devised by Dr Kenneth Cooper, needs only an accurately measured distance of 1.5 miles (a running track is ideal) and a stop watch. Having warmed up thoroughly, all you have to do is to cover the 1.5 miles as quickly as possible, noting the time it takes to run/jog the total distance. You can then compare your score using the table given (*Fig 3*). Like all running tests, this test will be influenced by your running technique, pace judgement, the weather conditions and even the running surface. Yet if the test is repeated under similar conditions on a regular basis, it will give you a reasonably good indication of aerobic fitness improvement.

Other simple tests of aerobic fitness rely upon the fact that during less than maximal exercise, like steady walking, cycling and stepping, an individual's heart rate increases as oxygen uptake increases. This makes it possible to measure a person's heart rate response to a given workload and predict with reasonable accuracy their maximal oxygen

Age (years)	very poor	poor	fair	good	very good	excellent	superb
Men							
17 – 29	16.30 +	14.30 +	12.00 +	10.15 +	8.15 +	7.30 +	6.45 +
30 – 34	17.00 +	15.00 +	12.30 +	10.30 +	8.30 +	7.45 +	7.00 +
35 – 39	17.30 +	15.30 +	13.00 +	10.45 +	8.45 +	8.00 +	7.15 +
40 – 44	18.00 +	16.00 +	13.30 +	11.00 +	9.00 +	8.15 +	7.30 +
45 – 49	18.30 +	16.30 +	14.00 +	11.15 +	9.15 +	8.30 +	7.45 +
over 50	19.00 +	17.00 +	14.30 +	11.30 +	9.30 +	8.45 +	8.00 +
Women							
17 – 29	19.48 +	17.24 +	14.24 +	12.18 +	9.54 +	9.00 +	8.06 +
30 – 34	20.24 +	18.00 +	15.00 +	12.36 +	10.12 +	9.18 +	8.24 +
35 – 39	21.00 +	18.36 +	15.36 +	12.54 +	10.30 +	9.36 +	8.42 +
40 – 44	21.36 +	19.12 +	16.12 +	13.12 +	10.48 +	9.54 +	9.00 +
45 – 49	22.12 +	19.48 +	16.48 +	13.30 +	11.06 +	10.30 +	9.36 +
over 50	22.48 +	20.24 +	17.24 +	13.48 +	11.24 +	10.30 +	9.36 +

Fig 3   Scoring table for the Cooper 1.5 mile run.

uptake, and hence their aerobic fitness. Such tests are now becoming increasingly available commercially: the Fitech Step Test is one such example. This kit comprises a cassette tape, booklet and calculator, you provide the step-up box (or stairs). Stepping up and down to the beat on the cassette for a given time, you then take your heart rate. This, along with your age and sex is plugged into the calculator and your fitness rating is given. Another similar system developed for the National Coaching Foundation is known as the Multi-Stage Fitness Test. This kit also contains a cassette and full instructions and requires you to run at a steadily increasing pace between two markers. The stage at which you can no longer keep pace with the cassette is noted, and referred to a table to give your fitness rating. Both systems are cheap and accurate.

More expensive systems require you to exercise on an accurate exercise bike and monitor your heart rate using some form of heart rate monitor. Again, these monitors are also becoming increasingly more commercially available. However, some of the monitors are more accurate than others. If you are going to purchase a heart rate monitor either to help you assess your aerobic fitness, or to work out how hard you are exercising (see Chapter 5) make sure that it attaches to your chest, rather than your finger or ear. The latter models tend to be less accurate. Some electronic exercise bikes (the expensive ones) also have built in computer programs which allow you to perform a fitness test using their built-in heart rate monitors, but their accuracy is questionable.

Unless you are prepared to calibrate your

exercise bike on a regular basis (to make sure the workload depicted is accurate) and purchase a good quality heart rate monitor, the simple aerobic fitness tests (1.5 mile run, Multi-Stage Fitness Test) are the best bet. They are accurate enough for most purposes, simple to do and cheap.

ASSESSING MUSCULAR STRENGTH AND ENDURANCE

The health-related components of fitness, muscular strength and muscular endurance are often confused with one another, yet the distinction between them is a clear one. Muscular strength reflects the amount of force that a muscle or muscle group can produce in overcoming a resistance, usually in one maximum, voluntary contraction (as in lifting a heavy weight), whilst muscular endurance reflects the ability of a muscle or muscle group to exert force repeatedly (as in lifting a light weight many times).

As with assessments of cardio-respiratory endurance, tests for gauging strength or endurance vary from the highly complex to the very simple. Some tests require sophisticated equipment costing many thousands of pounds. Such equipment (Cybex being a popular brand) makes it possible to evaluate accurately dynamic muscle strength, endurance, power, muscle imbalances and strength ratios. Other evaluation procedures, on the other hand, require simple equipment at most and even no equipment whatsoever. A common method of assessing strength which involves only one piece of equipment, which is popular in health clubs, involves the use of what is known as a handgrip dynamometer. This device is used to test the strength of the forearm flexors, and is a very simple test to administer. However, equally effective perhaps, and simpler still, is a test which is known as a 'timed sit-up'. This is a test of both muscular strength and endurance, and as its names suggests, is simply a measure of how many sit-ups an individual can perform in a given time period, usually 30 seconds. This test has been used extensively in a variety of situations and is employed for reasons other than its obvious simplicity. Many researchers feel that testing the condition of the abdominal muscles is most relevant to everyday life since these muscles are of vital importance in good posture and the prevention of back pain.

To perform the test, the person to be tested needs to lie on the floor with knees bent at right angles, feet comfortably apart and with their arms folded across the chest (*Fig 4*). The person performing the test holds the subject's

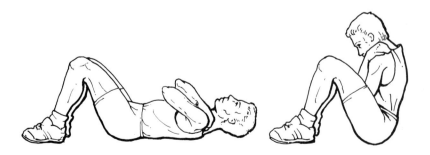

Fig 4   The timed sit-up test of muscular strength and endurance.

SCORING TABLE FOR THE TIMED SIT-UP TEST		
Rating	20 – 39 years	40 – 59 years
Poor	less than 17	less than 12
Fair	17 – 19	12 – 15
Average	20 – 21	16 – 17
Good	22 – 23	18 – 19
Excellent	24 or more	20 or more

Fig 5

ankles down so that both feet are kept firmly in contact with the floor at all times. Upon a signal from the tester, the subject curls up off the floor so that his/her elbows touch his/her thighs, and then curls down again. As soon as the subject's mid-back touches the floor, the movement sequence is repeated. The subject should breathe out as they curl up, and breathe in as they curl down. After 30 seconds the tester stops the test, having counted the exact number of completed curl ups performed in this time. Scores can then be compared with the table above (Fig 5).

ASSESSING FLEXIBILITY

The measurement of flexibility, or one's range of motion, may also be performed in a number of ways. In the laboratory it is common to use a device which is known as a 'Leighton Flexometer' and a series of accurately docu-mented tests which assess the range of motion at all the major joints from neck through to ankle. Naturally, these tests are time consuming and require the skills of a highly trained operator. Far simpler is an assessment procedure which is known as the 'sit-and-reach test'. Essentially this test is an assessment of lower back and hamstring flexibility, which is often used as an indicator of general joint and muscle mobility, and requires only simple equipment which can be made at home.

You will need a box and a ruler for the sit-and-reach test. Fix the ruler to the top of the box with clear tape, so that half of the ruler projects over the edge of the box. Now warm up thoroughly and sit with your bare feet placed against this side of the box, legs straight (Fig 6). Reach as far forward as possible with outstretched fingers (without bouncing) and note how far along the ruler your fingertips

SCORING TABLE FOR THE SIT-AND-REACH TEST	
Excellent	+ 15 cm
Good	+ 10 cm
Fair	+ 5 cm
Average	0 cm
Poor	less than 0 cm

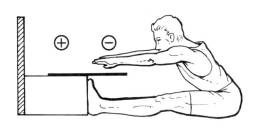

Fig 6   The sit-and-reach test of flexibility.

Fig 7

are. Distances past the edge of the box should be recorded as 'plus' values, whilst distances in front of the box should be recorded as 'minus' values. Compare your score on the best of three attempts with the following table (*Fig 7*).

ASSESSING
BODY COMPOSITION

The component of physical fitness known as body composition essentially reflects the 'make-up' of the body in terms of its relative percentages of muscle, fat, bone and other tissues. It is useful to know your body composition for a number of reasons. Initially from a health point of view, being over-fat is one of the main underlying causes of heart disease, hypertension and diabetes. Knowing your body composition allows you to know exactly whether you are over-fat or not. Traditionally it has been common to look at a person's weight and relate it to their height, subsequently arriving at a judgement as to whether they are overweight or not. Yet such a simple procedure says very little about how

---

Name: . . . . Age: . . . . Height: . . . . Weight: . . . . Date: . . . .

Girth measurements:
Upper arm: . . . . Chest/bust: . . . Waist: . . . . Hips: . . . . Upper thigh: . . Calf: . . . .

Aerobic fitness (1½ mile run test)   rating: . . . .
        or (Multi-stage fitness test)
        or (Step test)

Muscular endurance and strength test (Timed sit-up test)   rating: . . . .

Flexibility (Sit-and-reach test)   rating: . . . .

Comments on appearance and posture: . . . .

. . . .

. . . .

. . . .

. . . .

(N.B. When taking girth measurements, always ensure that you are measuring girths at the same site.)

Fig 8   Self-assessment record card.

much of that person's body is lean tissue and how much is fat, which is what really needs to be known as far as health is concerned. Knowing your body composition also allows you to observe the effectiveness of your exercise programme in helping you to change your shape and appearance.

Direct methods of estimating body composition, as with the other components of fitness, require sophisticated, expensive techniques. The simplest and cheapest method which can be carried out involves taking measurements of skinfold thicknesses at a variety of sites using specially designed callipers and/or circumference measurements. The basis for taking such measurements to assess body composition is a simple one: approximately 50 per cent of the body's total fat content lies just under the skin. Using this fact, measurements from pre-determined skinfold sites, and the appropriate formula, body composition can be simply computed. Obviously such an assessment needs practice and a strict attention to detail if reproducible results are to be obtained, yet simple kits, comprising callipers, tables and full instructions are readily purchased at small cost, and are probably a good investment.

Having completed a battery of health-related fitness tests such as those given above, you will now have a good idea of your initial fitness level. Use a chart, such as that given in *Fig 8,* to log the results of your assessment and note the date on which you carried out the tests. You will also see that there is room to record other measurements (weight, height, limb girths, etc.), which will further enable you to observe changes in your body brought about through exercise. Having recorded your results, you can now see at a glance which components of physical fitness are in most need of improvement. For instance, if your aerobic fitness rating is 'poor', whilst your other scores are 'good', you know that you need to concentrate upon this component in particular. The information in Chapter 5 (Exercise for Aerobic Fitness) will now tell you exactly how to go about this, just as Chapters 6 and 7 explain how to improve muscular strength, muscular endurance and flexibility.

Knowing your initial fitness level and having an idea as to which components of fitness you need to work upon in particular is essential, for reasons which have already been discussed. Yet if you are to exercise on a regular basis, the exercise activity you choose has to be something that you actually enjoy doing. You will find that the exercise programmes given for the various components of fitness in Chapters 5, 6 and 7 list many options and numerous ways of combining activities to achieve the specific goals you have in mind, so you should have no worries about becoming bored. The next step now in your fitness programme is to know how to put your individual programme together. This is explained in the next chapter.

3 Structuring an Exercise Programme

There is no secret formula when it comes to getting results from any exercise programme: all you have to do is follow a few simple rules which hold true no matter which components of fitness you are trying to improve. These rules basically reflect how the body responds to training. In the first instance it needs to be appreciated that the human body is dynamic, that is how it looks − and is − today, is different to how it will look and be tomorrow, or in a month's time. Things are constantly changing: cells are dying and being replaced by others. This remodelling of the body occurs throughout your lifetime at quicker or slower rates, with the rate of change being influenced by what is happening both inside and outside it. Some things are out of our immediate control: the ageing process will always occur, for example. However, the rate of functional decline associated with the ageing process can be slowed down through regular exercise, as indicated in Chapter 1, since physical activity improves physical function. This dynamic nature of the body is further illustrated by comparing tissues from active and inactive people. If you were to look at a muscle which is always active for example, you would see that it contains less fat than inactive muscle, has a greater blood supply, has more of the protein which causes it to contract, and has more stored energy. Similarly, a person who is aerobically active has a stronger heart, a greater network of blood vessels, more oxygen-carrying blood cells and even more blood than a similar person who is inactive. Yet if the active person were to become inactive for a period of time, his/her muscles and systems of the body would gradually assume the characteristics of inactive muscles and systems. All these adaptive changes, and more besides, occur in response to what the body is required to do. In other words, they occur as a result of the demands, or stress, placed upon the body.

When you exercise, or engage in some form of physical activity, you are basically asking the body to do more work than it does normally in the resting situation. Being highly adaptive, the body can react in the short term to meet these increased demands. So, during aerobic exercise, heart rate and breathing frequency will increase in an effort to supply more oxygen-rich blood to the working muscles. If the exercise bout is repeated, often enough, the body begins a more long-term adaptation. As mentioned, regular exercisers have more blood and more oxygen-carrying blood cells than non-exercisers. These adaptations mean that the body is better able to deliver oxygen to working muscles. In other words, the body is now more efficient when under physical stress, and what used to be hard work, is now easy because of these physiological changes.

Such adaptations within the body point to the first major training rule. In order to get any adaptation within the body and how it functions, you need to ask the body to do more work than it does normally. This training rule is often known as the principle of overload.

Yet achieving the right degree of overload is

crucial. Ask the body to do too much, and the results could be catastrophic. At the very least, you will suffer extreme muscle soreness, and may even be on the receiving end of some more acute injury, like a torn muscle or ruptured tendon. At the worst, too much exercise of too high an intensity can even cause a heart attack in susceptible individuals. (Fortunately, such instances are rare). Correspondingly, too little overload means that no adaptation occurs, and from a physiological point of view, you might as well not be exercising at all!

To achieve the right amount of overload, you need to consider a few other factors. Your initial fitness level obviously. This you now know, having performed the reasonably detailed fitness assessment which was given in the previous chapter. Basically, the less fit you are, the smaller the total overload necessary to achieve a training effect, and incidentally, the more rapidly the observable benefits of exercise will occur. Thirty to forty minutes a day, three times a week for the very unfit will bring about noticeable results in a few weeks, for example. Olympic athletes, on the other hand, will find themselves training for many hours a day just to see small improvements in performance over a period of months, or even years.

The next point you need to consider is exactly why you are exercising. Answering this question then allows you to decide upon the type of exercise you are going to do; the intensity and duration of that exercise, and how often you are going to repeat that exercise bout. To give an example, if you are aiming to increase muscular strength, you need to do some type of resistance exercise. Furthermore, the resistance exercise in question needs to be of high intensity, and will correspondingly be of short duration. The exercise bout will need to be repeated with a frequency of about four times a week. Detailed programmes for the development of

any component of fitness can be found in the appropriate chapter, and such simple rules can be outlined for all training aims, since all training programmes whatever and whoever they are for, simply manipulate these variables to get the most appropriate training overload.

Finally, carrying out a particular type of exercise, at a particular intensity, for a specific duration with a specific frequency means that you are doing a given amount of physical work in your training session. All being well, your body will adapt to that training load over a period of time. Having adapted, that training load is no longer suitable to cause any further change in the body. You will now maintain fitness if you keep doing the same amount of work, but you will not improve. Further adaptations, and hence further improvement, now means that you will have to increase the workload again. This may mean increasing either the intensity of the exercise, its duration, its frequency or even all three, depending upon your reasons for exercising. This is the final golden rule as far as exercise is concerned: all exercise programmes, if they are to achieve continuing benefits, must be progressive in nature.

Structuring any exercise programme to follow these rules is a fairly simple, logical process. It is made simpler still by ordering your training programme, just as Olympic athletes do, so that you have set aims as the weeks go by, and you make a regular note of your progress and how you feel, using a training diary. This need only be a simple notebook. An example of a training log is shown in *Fig 9*, which should make it easy to keep a general record.

If you wish to record specific information about a particular activity, like weight training, for example, structure a record card similar to the one shown in *Fig 10* to outline your session. It is not necessary to use a fresh record card every time you train, just when you change your training in some way.

21

Date	Session	Type of training	Intensity	Duration	Comments

Fig 9   Your training log.

Having decided which exercise activities you are going to do, and what type of a programme you are going to follow (from your fitness assessment, your personal preferences and the information given in the exercise chapters), you should start your training programme, with the first training session labelled as 'day 1'. (Add 'session 1', etc., if you intend to exercise twice in one day). Each training session should contain warm-up and warm-down (see Chapter 4) phases which will sandwich the training phase proper. Write down everything you do in this training phase, as indicated in Appendix 1. Do this for every training session, so that at the end of your training week you know exactly what you have done. If certain aspects of the training get easier, observe this in the 'comments' section, and adjust your exercise programme accordingly the following week. At the end of 10 to 12 weeks of progressive training, repeat your fitness assessment. Now you can assess the effectiveness of your training programme and adjust it accordingly, perhaps with

different training aims in mind. Repeat this process every 10 to 12 weeks, noting your improvement each time through a repeat assessment.

The only other important points as far as structuring your exercise programme goes relate to avoiding injury. Certainly you should never exercise at all if you feel unwell, or if you have a virus or any other medical condition you are unsure about. Neither should you exercise if you have an injury of any sort, or if you have been drinking alcoholic beverages. Likewise, you should not exercise following a heavy meal. Generally speaking, you need to allow approximately two to three hours to digest a heavy meal before engaging in vigorous physical activity.

If whilst you are exercising you feel at all unwell, stop exercising and get specialist advice. Sensations of dizziness and nausea may only mean that you are exercising too vigorously, particularly if these sensations are accompanied by skin pallor or unsteadiness. If they occur more than once, or you do not

Session No:	Week no:	Date:		
Exercise (E) or Recovery (R)	Weight	Repetitions	Time	Work load (Weight × repetitions)
E				
R				
E				
R				
E				
R				
E				
R				
E				
R				
E				
R				
E				
R				
E				
R				
E				
R				
E				
R				
E				
R				
E				
R				
E				
R				
E				
R				
E				
R		Total		

Number of circuits:

Comments:

Fig 10   Record card.

recover quickly from these sensations, see your GP. Pain is also a sign that something is wrong, especially if that pain is sudden. Sudden pains invariably indicate injury. Stop immediately and seek advice. Exercising through an injury will make the problem worse, any injury will take longer to heal and you may be unable to train properly for a long time. It is far better to seek early treatment and get back into full training sooner rather than later.

If you are exercising for the first time following a long time away from regular physical activity, it is not unusual to feel some stiffness and soreness a day or two after your first few exercise bouts. If this soreness or stiffness is so acute that you cannot perform another exercise bout two days later, you have been exercising at too great an intensity. Adjust your exercise session accordingly, and make sure that you warm up and warm down thoroughly.

4 Warming Up and Warming Down

Up until recently, warming up and warming down as part of an exercise session received scant mention. At best, most regular exercisers whirled their arms around a few times and shook their legs twice before launching into vigorous physical activity. At the end of the session, a couple of short stretches constituted the warm-down.

Nowadays, warming up and warming down are seen as essential and integral parts of any exercise routine, so much so, that for some people, these phases of the activity session last almost as long as the training phase itself. This new emphasis on these components of a training programme is largely because research has shown that preparing yourself properly for exercise (warming up), and recovering appropriately from any physical activity (warming down) offers many positive benefits.

A good warm-up routine has been shown to lead to all kinds of beneficial physiological changes. As the name of this phase suggests, a warm-up effectively increases the temperature of the body. This in turn leads to a number of observed benefits. To begin with, the increase in temperature of the body makes muscles less viscous, so that they can contract and relax more readily. Nerve impulses also find that they can travel more quickly and be received more easily. Increased body temperature also means that oxygen can be made more available to the muscles for energy processes, and that the chemical reactions which take part in these processes take place more efficiently. Studies on cardiac patients

have also shown that the response of the heart to sudden strenuous exercise is improved with a warm-up. Finally, warming up appropriately means that muscles, tendons and joint structures in general are less likely to be damaged once you start exercising.

Warming down following exercise allows the body to return back to normal quickly and efficiently. During strenuous exercise, the body shunts blood around the body to where it is most needed, namely to the working muscles. It is not uncommon, for example, for a working muscle to increase its blood flow 20-fold during very vigorous exercise. If you stop still after such vigorous activity, blood has a tendency to 'pool' in the extremities, particularly in the muscles of the lower body. This necessarily means that less blood is flowing to other vital parts of the body, like the brain, hence the feelings of dizziness. You can prevent this, and help the body to recover more quickly, by gradually decreasing the intensity of your exercise. Keeping the muscles working in light, rhythmical movements effectively pumps the blood back to the heart allowing the body rapidly to return to normal. A comprehensive stretching sequence carried out now, whilst the body is very warm indeed also seems to help prevent muscle soreness, as well as dramatically increasing your range of movement.

There are a number of methods of warming up, but what all methods are basically trying to do is increase the temperature of the body, and take the muscles and joints of the body through as full a range of movement as possible. The most commonly recommended method is known as a 'dynamic warm-up'. To begin with, you need to dress warmly, preferably in several layers of clothing which can easily be removed. You then need to carry out some form of light, rhythmical activity which involves large muscle groups – stationary cycling, for example. As muscles produce movement they also generate a massive amount of heat which is carried around the body by the blood. This is soon noticed as you cycle at an easy pace and the layers of clothing insulate you and prevent the generated heat being lost to the air. In the space of a few minutes most people will find themselves feeling much warmer and perspiring slightly. You then need to carry out some general joint mobilisers such as those given in the sample warm-up section. These exercises ensure that your muscles and joints have gone through their normal ranges of movement prior to more vigorous activity. Finally, a few preparatory stretches for muscles groups which will feature heavily in the main exercise phase will prevent injury. Instructions for the stretching exercises themselves are given in Chapter 7, and the sample preparatory stretching programme is given at the end of the warm-up exercises.

The length of a warm-up phase will vary according to fitness, the exercise you are about to do, age, and environmental conditions. The older or the more unfit you are, generally the longer you should spend warming up. Ten minutes should suffice most people, however. If it is particularly warm, your muscles are also likely to be warm, hence you may only need to do some general mobility work and preparatory stretching, dispensing with the large muscle group work altogether. If you are planning a very strenuous work out, spend more time than normal warming up. Obviously, remove any layers of clothing you are wearing to prevent yourself from becoming excessively hot.

Warming down is also easily done. As indicated, gradually decrease the intensity of your exercise phase. If you have been running, for example, at the end of your run, jog easily for a few minutes. Replace any layers of clothing you may have removed as you became warmer earlier on in your exercise session, and then repeat the mobilising exercises given in the sample warm-up phase. Finish off with a comprehensive sequence of developmental stretches. Different stretching programmes you may like to choose from for this final stage of your exercise phase are listed in Chapter 7.

WARMING UP EXERCISES

The first part of your warm-up phase involves an aerobic large muscle group activity. This can take many forms and largely depends upon your personal preferences and the availability of equipment. Any of the exercises listed in the chapter dealing with aerobic fitness (Chapter 5) can be employed in this section, for example. Whichever activity you choose, it should be of low intensity and feel easy. To give an example, if you were to choose stationary cycling as your warming up activity, pedalling at a frequency of around 70 crank revolutions per minute (see *Fig 25* in Chapter 5) with no resistance for a couple of minutes is an ideal start. After these first two minutes, you can then add a minimum of resistance, whilst keeping the pedalling frequency the same, for a further three minutes. You will then have completed a total of five minutes of easy activity, will be somewhat warmer and ready to carry out the mobilising exercises given here. Advice about using any other aerobic activity for warming up is further outlined in Chapter 5.

The exercises given here as mobilisers are just a sample of what you might like to do.

Other exercises can be used equally effectively in this phase as long as they take muscles and joints through a full range of movement in a rhythmical manner. If using other exercises, try and organise them so that the exercises which involve the largest muscle groups are carried out first.

Throughout these exercises, and others which feature in later sections of the book, the instructions will often tell you to 'stand (or sit) with good posture'. This means that you should be aiming for a balanced head, long neck, shoulders back and down away from your ears, long spine and centrally balanced pelvis. If standing, feet should be about shoulder-width apart. Exercising with good posture makes all the movements and exercises that much more effective and you should therefore aim for good posture at all times in your exercise programme.

(Perform all exercises one after the other. Do not bounce, jerk or force yourself into any position).

1. Half Squat (*Fig 11*)

Stand tall with good posture. Rest your hands on your hips, or hold them out in front of you for balance. Now bend at the knees until your thighs are parallel to the floor. Keep your back long throughout the movement, look straight ahead and make sure that your knees always point in the same direction as your toes. Once at your lowest point, fully straighten your legs to return to your starting position. Breathe in as you descend, and breathe out as you rise. Repeat the exercise sixteen times with a smooth, even rhythm.

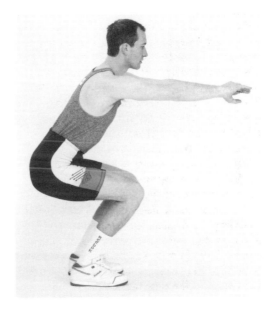

Fig 11   Half squat.

2. Knees to Chest (*Fig 12*)

Stand tall with good posture. Keeping your body upright, bring one knee up towards your chest to meet the elbow of the opposite arm. Repeat with the opposite arm and leg, and then repeat the whole sequence sixteen times, breathing easily throughout.

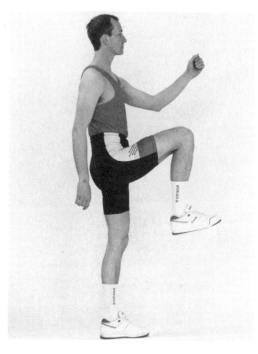

Fig 12   Knees to chest.

3. Bench Stepping (*Fig 13*)

Stand tall with good posture in front of a strong, stable bench or stool. Step onto the bench with one foot, straightening this leg fully to stand tall on the bench. Step down with the other leg. Repeat the exercise sixteen times, then change the leading leg and repeat a further sixteen times, maintaining a smooth, even rhythm. Breathe comfortably throughout the exercise.

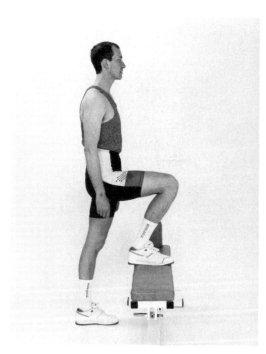

Fig 13   Bench stepping.

4. Side Bends
(Fig 14)

Stand tall with good posture. Have your feet slightly wider than shoulder-width apart and bend your knees slightly, resting your hands on your hips. Lift your trunk up and away from your hips and bend smoothly first to one side, then the other, avoiding the tendency to lean either forwards or backwards. Repeat the whole sequence sixteen times, breathing out as you bend to the side, and in as you return to the centre.

5. Shoulder Circles
(Fig 15)

Stand tall with good posture. Raise your right shoulder towards your right ear, take it backwards, then down and up again in a circular motion. Repeat eight times with a smooth rhythm. Continue with the other shoulder. Breathe easily throughout the sequence.

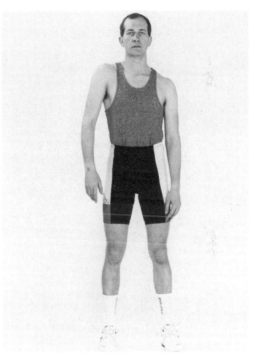

Fig 15   Shoulder circles.

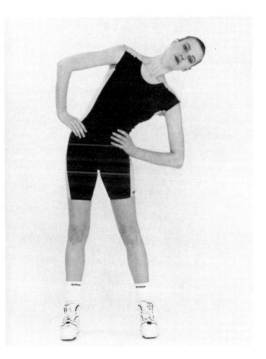

Fig 14   Side bends.

6. Arm Circles
(*Fig 16*)

Stand tall with good posture. Lift one arm forward then take it backwards in a continuous circling motion, keeping your spine long throughout. Repeat eight times, then perform the exercise with the other arm. Avoid the tendency to arch your back. Breathe easily throughout the sequence.

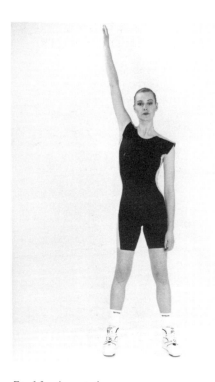

Fig 16 Arm circles.

These mobilisers cover the major joints and muscle groups. As mentioned earlier, there are other options, using other free-standing exercises like these, or even using equipment. For example, if you have purchased a home gym, or some weights, and resistance training is going to be your training activity for that session, you can carry out a general resistance training circuit, as outlined in Chapter 6, but using very light weights, before continuing with your preparatory stretching. You can also use exercises 1, 2 and 3 as a whole-body warm-up rather than the aerobic activities outlined in Chapter 5. To do this, merely repeat these exercises in sequence a total of three times (i.e. three circuits) before moving on to exercises, 4, 5 and 6.

The next phase of your warm-up is the preparatory stretching. A full range of stretching exercises and instructions on how to carry them out safely is given in Chapter 7. Preparatory stretches need only be held for 6 seconds, as opposed to around 30 seconds for developmental stretches and a sample general preparatory stretching sequence is given on pages 31–2 in Fig 17.

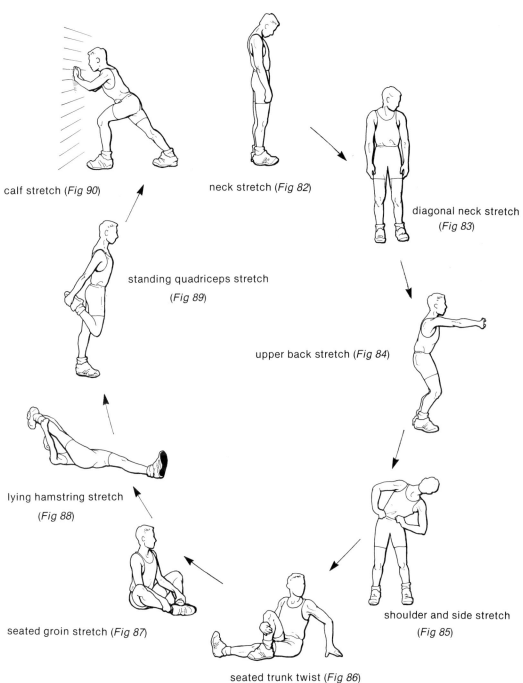

calf stretch (*Fig 90*)

neck stretch (*Fig 82*)

diagonal neck stretch
(*Fig 83*)

standing quadriceps stretch
(*Fig 89*)

upper back stretch (*Fig 84*)

lying hamstring stretch
(*Fig 88*)

seated groin stretch (*Fig 87*)

seated trunk twist (*Fig 86*)

shoulder and side stretch
(*Fig 85*)

Fig 17   Preparatory stretching sequence.

PREPARATORY STRETCHING SEQUENCE

Perform the following stretches. The numbers refer to the exercises described in Chapter 7, and you should follow the exercise instructions given in this chapter, holding each stretch for approximately 6 seconds.

Neck stretch	(*Fig 82*)
Diagonal neck stretch	(*Fig 83*)
Upper back stretch	(*Fig 84*)
Shoulder and side stretch	(*Fig 85*)
Seated trunk twist	(*Fig 86*)
Seated groin stretch	(*Fig 87*)
Lying hamstring stretch	(*Fig 88*)
Standing quadriceps stretch	(*Fig 89*)
Calf stretch	(*Fig 90*)

Having warmed up thoroughly, you are now ready to continue with the training phase of your exercise session, safe in the knowledge that your body is fully prepared and raring to go.

Fig 17

5 Exercise for Aerobic Fitness

For any exercise to be considered aerobic, as has already been stated, it must use large muscle groups in rhythmical contractions (in other words, the muscles in question must contract and relax on a regular basis). Further, the exercise should make you comfortably out of breath and should be capable of being performed, continuously, for several minutes. All the activities in this chapter can meet those criteria, and may be chosen, according to individual preference and availability of equipment, to improve your aerobic fitness rating.

The exact intensity that an aerobic activity should be performed at, and its duration, depend largely upon your initial fitness level and your reasons for exercising. As pointed out in Chapter 3, the less fit you are, the lower the intensity and the smaller the overload necessary to elicit a training effect. Strictly speaking, the intensity of aerobic exercise should be assessed relative to an individual's maximum oxygen uptake ($\dot{V}O_2$max). Yet because of the inaccessibility of such measurements in the normal exercising situation, a more convenient method of assessing exercise intensity is to monitor your heart rate, and work at a percentage of predicted maximum heart rate. This procedure is valid during aerobic exercise, since the increase in heart rate observed whilst exercising aerobically reflects the increase in $\dot{V}O_2$ max. A standard technique for working out maximum predicted heart rate, and exercise heart rates, is shown in *Fig 18*.

ASSESSING YOUR MAXIMUM HEART RATE

During aerobic exercise, the harder you work, the faster your heart beats. As your heart beats, the blood vessels expand and contract as blood is pumped through them: this is what produces your pulse.

Your pulse can be easily located at several sites. The two most common sites for taking your pulse are at the carotid artery in the neck and the radial artery in the wrist.

How to Find Your Carotid Pulse

If you are right-handed, find your carotid pulse using the first two fingers of your right hand, placed against the left-hand side of the neck just below the jaw bone. Apply light finger pressure only. Pressing too hard can cause a reflex slowing of the heart.

How to Find Your Radial Pulse

If you are right-handed, find your radial pulse using the first two fingers of your right hand placed on the thumb side of your left wrist. Again, apply light finger pressure only.

Having located your pulse at either site, start counting the number of pulses over a 10-second interval. The first beat you count is zero, then one, two, three . . . etc. Having counted the number of beats in 10 seconds, multiply this figure by six to find your heart rate in beats per minute. If the number of beats is, say, 12 in 10 seconds, then $12 \times 6 = 72$ beats per minute.

The best time to take your resting pulse is first thing in the morning, as you awake and before your body has had to do anything which might raise your heart rate above its normal resting value. Remember that higher than normal pulse rates can be caused by stimulants like tea, coffee, certain soft drinks and nicotine, as well as by emotional stress, fatigue and illness or injury.

The best time to take your exercise heart rate is naturally, during exercise. This is difficult manually, and most people find that they have to stop exercising in order to count accurately. In this situation, try and keep large muscle groups, such as those in the legs moving lightly and rhythmically and locate, and count your pulse as quickly as possible, since heart rate falls rapidly from its exercise level.

Your maximum predicted heart rate can be gauged by subtracting your age in years from the number 220. So, if you are thirty years old, your predicted maximum heart rate will be $220 - 30 = 190$ beats per minute. Knowing

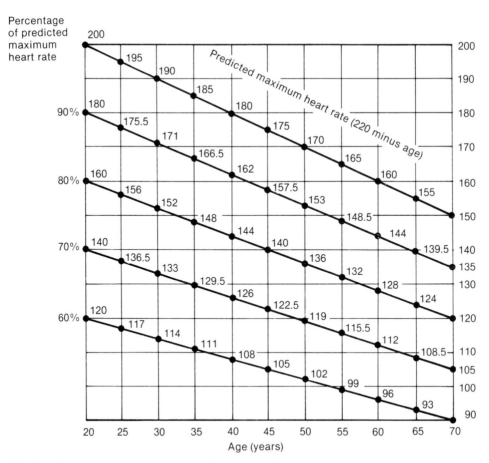

Fig 18 Estimating predicted maximum heart rate and percentages.

your predicted maximum heart rate enables you to calculate percentages of your maximum which will allow you to work at the correct exercise intensity according to your aims and fitness level. *Fig 18* sets out the predicted maximum heart rates according to age, and also percentages of the maximum. This enables you to read off what your heart rate should be relative to exercise intensity.

It doesn't actually take that long for you to know just how hard you are working, once you have monitored your heart rate a few times during different activities carried out at different intensities. However, to be more certain of what your exercise heart rate really is, you will need to purchase a heart-rate monitor. As indicated in Chapter 2, the best heart-rate monitors for home use are those which have chest electrodes and can be easily attached to a belt, for instance. There are many varieties currently available and whilst such devices may seem to be extravagant as far as some people are concerned, they are very useful if you are training with a view to improving sports performance and wish to mimic the demands of your performance activity. More expensive heart rate monitors also record your heart rate throughout the whole of an exercise bout.

Traditionally, to improve your aerobic fitness, it has been recommended that you should exercise at greater than 50 per cent of your maximum oxygen uptake, which is equivalent to approximately 60 per cent of maximum heart rate. Yet it has been shown more recently that people who have never exercised before, or who follow a sedentary lifestyle can train at intensities as low as 40 per cent VO_2 max (50 per cent MHR) and still achieve a training effect. It has also been shown that there is no great advantage, if any at all, to be gained by exercising at greater than 90 per cent VO_2 max. Indeed, the risk of injury escalates disproportionally with an increase in exercise intensity. For general

fitness benefits, aerobic exercise needs to be of an intensity of between 40–70 per cent VO_2 max (50–85 per cent MHR). The less fit should concentrate their exercise at the lower end of this scale, as indeed should those people who are interested in exercising with a view to fat loss. Body fat can be used as fuel for exercise in significant quantities, only if the exercise is continuous and of relatively low intensity, (50 per cent VO_2 max/60 per cent MHR), and of long duration (20 minutes plus). Sportsmen and athletes may, however, have to exercise at higher intensities, as will fitter individuals, yet the exact intensity necessary to achieve the required training effect will depend upon individual fitness and upon the event/sport, and is best decided by the performer's coach or training adviser.

Exercise duration depends, once again, upon the training aim, initial fitness level and exercise intensity. For general fitness benefits, anywhere between 30 and 60 minutes (depending upon fitness) of aerobic exercise of moderate intensity as indicated, repeated 3–4 times a week will bring excellent results. If your training aim is fat loss, then you will have to keep to low intensity exercise and extend its duration to a 40 minutes minimum 3–4 times a week.

It is also possible to improve aerobic fitness through bouts of higher intensity aerobic exercise (75–85 per cent VO_2 max), of short duration (5–10 minutes) separated by a short (5–10 minutes) recovery phase of low intensity (up to 40 per cent VO_2 max) aerobic exercise. This type of aerobic conditioning is known as 'Interval Aerobics', and because of its very demanding nature should only be carried out by the very well-conditioned in the first place.

It should be clear now, that there are many ways of conditioning the body through aerobic activities, just through varying the programmes alone, with each type of programme bringing slightly different training

TRAINING AIMS AND EXERCISE INTENSITY		
Aim	**Intensity** (as a percentage of HR)	**Duration**
to use body fat as fuel for the activity	50 – 60%	40 minutes plus
to generally improve the aerobic system	50 – 85% (according to fitness)	30 minutes +
interval aerobics	80 – 90%	5 – 10 minutes (repeated)

Fig 19

benefits. This information is summarised in table form in *Fig 19*.

It is also possible to get slightly different training effects according to which aerobic activities you use. Whilst the cardio-respiratory changes associated with different activities performed at the same relative intensity are largely the same, different activities will produce different local effects according to which muscles and joints are used, and how they are used. The different benefits of each aerobic activity are listed in the appropriate activity section in this chapter. Note that it is possible to combine aerobic activities to achieve a total aerobic conditioning effect, or to make aerobic training more varied and perhaps more interesting, as indicated at the end of this chapter in *Fig 34*, and also in Chapter 9.

AEROBIC ACTIVITIES

1. Walking

In Great Britain, the Sports Council have estimated that walking for pleasure and recreation is one of the country's most popular activities, being regularly carried out by approximately 22 per cent of the adult population (around 9.5 million people). Many experts are also of the opinion that walking is one of the most underrated fitness activities, perhaps because it seems so easy to do. Yet walking at a brisk pace on a regular basis can improve aerobic fitness substantially, especially if you are relatively unfit, and walking can serve as an introduction to other aerobic activities which may need a higher level of aerobic fitness than you currently possess if they are to be enjoyed.

Walking for fitness is also a good idea for the heavily overweight, since it does not involve high impact forces. In other words, the force with which your foot hits the floor with each step is low. It has been estimated that running, for example, produces impact forces with each stride which are approximately three times your body weight. The impact forces which occur during walking are, however, only one third of this. This means that the injury risk associated with walking is low, making the activity very suitable for the very unfit, the elderly and even post-operative cardiac patients, as well as the overweight.

If you are still not convinced, noted exercise researcher Ralph Paffenbarger has shown that walking an average of nine miles per week throughout one's lifetime significantly reduces the likelihood of developing heart disease. Further, walking requires little specialist equipment, other than comfortable clothing and a good pair of walking shoes.

Fitness walking needs to be brisk and is not a dawdle, stopping to look in shop windows, and you should be aiming to cover three miles an hour. Walk with a good full stride, pushing firmly off the back leg and cultivate a feeling of walking tall. Arms should swing loosely by your sides, and if you need to carry anything, purchase a small rucksack rather than have a bag slung over one shoulder. Walking can be made more demanding as you become fitter by carrying small hand weights and pumping your arms more: this is commonly known as 'Power Walking'. If you are going to do this, bear in mind that the weights used should be no more than 2kg each and should be gradually introduced into your programme. Injuries have been associated with Power Walking, mainly through the use of weights which were far too heavy. The programme in *Fig 20* is for beginners, and the accompanying information explains how to progress as your fitness improves.

Fig 20

BEGINNER'S WALKING PROGRAMME

The following 12-week programme assumes that you have been relatively inactive for some time. If you find you are progressing more quickly than the programme indicates, move ahead by an appropriate number of sessions, yet still follow the same basic rules.

Remember to warm up and warm down as indicated in the previous chapter.

At the end of this programme you will find that you are easily walking every other day for 45 minutes. This is a good level to stay at for general fitness benefits. If you wish to increase your total walking time over the next few weeks, do so, progressing in a similar fashion to that indicated here.

You can always increase the intensity of your walking programme if you wish, too. Try increasing the pace of one of your walks each week, say to 70 per cent MHR. If you find this uncomfortable, drop back to your normal intensity. If you feel that you are ready to go faster still, try the jogging programme in the next section.

Activity:	Walking			
Week 1	Intensity	Duration (mins)	Resistance setting	Pedal/stroke frequency
Day 1	60% MHR	20		
Day 3	60% MHR	20		
Day 5	60% MHR	20		
Day 7	60% MHR	20		

Week 2	Intensity	Duration (mins)	Resistance setting	Pedal/stroke frequency
Day 2	60% MHR	22		
Day 4	60% MHR	20		
Day 6	60% MHR	22		
Week 3				
Day 1	60% MHR	20		
Day 3	60% MHR	24		
Day 5	60% MHR	22		
Day 7	60% MHR	20		
Week 4				
Day 2	60% MHR	26		
Day 4	60% MHR	22		
Day 6	60% MHR	24		
Week 5				
Day 1	60% MHR	22		
Day 3	60% MHR	28		
Day 5	60% MHR	24		
Day 7	60% MHR	22		
Week 6				
Day 2	60% MHR	30		
Day 4	60% MHR	24		
Day 6	60% MHR	24		
Week 7				
Day 1	60% MHR	35		
Day 3	60% MHR	30		
Day 5	60% MHR	25		
Day 7	60% MHR	25		

Fig 20

Week 8	Intensity	Duration (mins)	Resistance setting	Pedal/stroke frequency
Day 2	60% MHR	30		
Day 4	60% MHR	40		
Day 6	60% MHR	30		
Week 9				
Day 1	60% MHR	35		
Day 3	60% MHR	40		
Day 5	60% MHR	30		
Day 7	60% MHR	35		
Week 10				
Day 2	60% MHR	40		
Day 4	60% MHR	45		
Day 6	60% MHR	40		
Week 11				
Day 1	60% MHR	30		
Day 3	60% MHR	45		
Day 5	60% MHR	30		
Day 7	60% MHR	45		
Week 12				
Day 2	60% MHR	45		
Day 4	60% MHR	45		
Day 6	60% MHR	45		

Fig 20

2. Jogging/Running

After walking for fitness, jogging and running are perhaps the next simplest activities to carry out as part of a home exercise programme. Again, little specialist equipment is needed, just comfortable clothing and appropriate shoes, and the fitness benefits associated with both activities are well documented. The differences between walking, jogging and running are mainly in technique and pace. Technically in walking for example, one foot is always in contact with the ground. This is not the case with jogging or running, however, since in both these activities there is an unsupported phase when both feet are off the ground: this is perhaps most obvious when watching sprinters. The other difference between the three activities is then one of speed. Fitness walkers will travel at a speed of around 3 m.p.h., joggers cover around 6 m.p.h. and runners will be travelling at 7 m.p.h. and faster.

Walking programmes form a firm basis for jogging programmes, which in turn provide the foundation for running. If you have never jogged or run for fitness before, start off with a walking programme as given earlier. As you become fitter you should incorporate more jogging, as indicated in the jogging programme given here. Once you are jogging comfortably and regularly, you can then start to think about speeding up if you want to, and a sample running programme is given, which follows on from the jogging programme given in *Fig 21*.

BEGINNER'S JOGGING PROGRAMME

The beginners' jogging programme given here assumes that you can cope relatively easily with the walking programme given earlier. It has also been designed to enable you, if you so wish, to enter a 10-kilometre fun run at the end of it. The key aspect of this programme, as with the walking programme is that the pace should be comfortable, and you should forget all about speed. Work intensely enough to take your heart rate to approximately 60 per cent of the maximum, but other than that, do not worry about how far or how fast you are going.

Once again, remember to warm up and warm down thoroughly.

Fig 21

Activity:	Jogging			
Week 1	Intensity	Duration (mins)	Resistance setting	Pedal/stroke frequency
Day 1	All runs at	20		
Day 3	60% MHR	20		
Day 5		20		
Day 7		20		

	Intensity	Duration (mins)	Resistance setting	Pedal/stroke frequency
Week 2				
Day 2		20		
Day 4		23		
Day 6		20		
Week 3				
Day 1		20		
Day 3		23		
Day 5		20		
Day 7		25		
Week 4				
Day 2		20		
Day 4		23		
Day 6		27		
Week 5				
Day 1		20		
Day 3		23		
Day 5		20		
Day 7		30		
Week 6				
Day 2		23		
Day 4		27		
Day 6		32		
Week 7				
Day 1		23		
Day 3		25		
Day 5		23		
Day 7		35		

Fig 21

Week 8	Intensity	Duration (mins)	Resistance setting	Pedal/stroke frequency
Day 2		25		
Day 4		27		
Day 6		37		
Week 9				
Day 1		27		
Day 3		23		
Day 5		30		
Day 7		40		
Week 10				
Day 2		30		
Day 4		27		
Day 6		45		
Week 11				
Day 1		25		
Day 3		35		
Day 5		27		
Day 7		50		
Week 12				
Day 2		27		
Day 4		35		
Day 6		55		

Fig 21

Once you are running regularly, you may then like to think about entering a fun run or general road race. Such events give you something to aim for and provide motivation and are great fun if you are the competitive type. You will also then find yourself mixing with other runners who will, no doubt, explain that there is more to running than just going at the same pace.

A beginner's running programme is outlined in *Fig 22*.

BEGINNER'S RUNNING PROGRAMME

Having worked through the previous walking and jogging programmes, you have now been doing some form of systematic aerobic training for six months. You will also have worked up to running at least five miles continuously at an even, steady, comfortable pace.

The running programme here shows how you can move up over the next three months to running longer distances if you wish, and aims to prepare you for a half marathon (13.1 miles). Naturally, you may not want to do this, but the following programme shows you how to structure your running programme so that you can run for longer.

Again, the intensity of the exercise is moderate: aim for an exercise heart rate of between 60 and 80 per cent of maximum.

Instead of time, this programme now looks at distance.

Fig 22

Activity:	Running			
Week 1	Intensity	Duration (miles)	Resistance setting	Pedal/stroke frequency
Day 1	All runs at	4		
Day 3	60% – 80%	5		
Day 5	MHR	4		
Day 7		5		

	Intensity	Duration (miles)	Resistance setting	Pedal/stroke frequency
Week 2				
Day 2		4		
Day 4		5		
Day 6		6		
Week 3				
Day 1		4		
Day 3		5		
Day 5		4		
Day 7		6		
Week 4				
Day 2		4		
Day 4		5		
Day 6		7		
Week 5				
Day 1		5		
Day 3		7		
Day 5		5		
Day 7		7		
Week 6				
Day 2		5		
Day 4		6		
Day 6		8		
Week 7				
Day 1		6		
Day 3		8		
Day 5		6		
Day 7		8		

Fig 22

Week 8	Intensity	Duration (miles)	Resistance setting	Pedal/stroke frequency
Day 2		5		
Day 4		9		
Day 6		6		
Week 9				
Day 1		6		
Day 3		9		
Day 5		5		
Day 7		10		
Week 10				
Day 2		5		
Day 4		6		
Day 6		10		
Week 11				
Day 1		6		
Day 3		8		
Day 5		5		
Day 7		11		
Week 12				
Day 2		6		
Day 4		5		
Day 6		13.1		

Fig 22

All walking, jogging and running programmes can be done indoors on a piece of
equipment which is called a treadmill or
running machine. Treadmills come in two
main varieties: motorised and non-motorised
(*Fig 23*). Non-motorised versions basically
consist of a frame and a series of rollers which
may or may not be covered by a belt. You
then walk, run or jog upon the rollers. Whilst
such machines are relatively cheap, the
action is poor and feels nothing like the real
thing. Motorised treadmills allow you to
replicate walking and running actions far more
accurately, but they are expensive. The
running surface is again a belt of some nature,
but this is driven by a motor. Most models
allow the belt to travel at speeds up to 20km
per hour, which is equivalent to a mile every

five minutes. Some versions also feature an
incline option, which may or may not be
motor driven. The most sophisticated models
also feature computer programs which you
can choose or design yourself, so that the
speed and incline varies as if you were running
over the countryside. Other machines allow
you to perform all types of interval training and
repetition running.

Motorised treadmills are a great alternative
to the real thing, and have been used with
great success by international runners living in
inclement climates who cannot run outside as
often as they would like, or need to. Their
main drawback as far as the home user is
concerned is one of finance, with even the
cheaper, no frills models costing upwards of
£2,000. If you can afford one, bear in mind
also that they do make quite a lot of noise,
especially at faster speeds. You will also find
that most models will need an operating space
of at least 2m × 1m. Finally, exercising on a
treadmill does mean that you will become very
hot, very quickly, since you will miss out on
the cooling effect which occurs as you run outside. A useful purchase to offset this problem is
a fan, which should be placed in front of your
treadmill.

Types of running training are outlined in *Fig
24*.

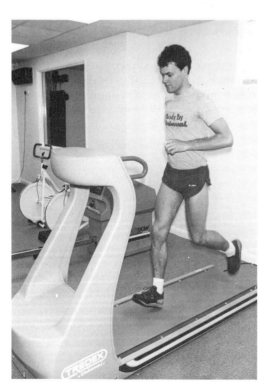

Fig 23   Computerised treadmill.

Types of running training

LONG, SLOW DISTANCE (LSD)

This is the type of running you have been doing if you have been following the beginnners' running programme given here. LSD refers to any type of running which is at the same pace and which essentially lasts over 30 minutes duration. Intensity of such running is light to moderate (between 60 and 80 per cent MHR). LSD running conditions the oxygen transporting systems of the body, makes muscles and joints stronger and more resistant to fatigue, and, as the distance increases, uses increasingly more fat as the fuel for running.

CONTINUOUS FAST RUNNING

As the intensity of a run increases, so the duration of the run will decrease. Continuous fast running demands that you work at a higher intensity than LSD running: approximately 85 per cent MHR. This type of training conditions the body to run at race pace or faster, and further strengthens the muscles and joints of the lower body.

FARTLEK RUNNING

If both fast and slow running are incorporated in the same training session according to how you feel and the terrain (hills, even ground, etc.) then this type of running training is known as fartlek. Intensity of fartlek running naturally varies from 60 per cent − 90 per cent MHR. An excellent way of combining the benefits of all types of running in one session.

INTERVAL TRAINING

Interval training is basically formalised fartlek running. After a bout of running there follows a bout of recovery. This is followed by another bout of running, then more recovery. This is repeated until the session is completed. Interval training can be used to develop speed, endurance, the aerobic system, the anaerobic system, according to how the interval training is structured.

Fig 24

3. Cycling

As far as home exercise goes, the stationary cycle is by far the most popular purchase in Great Britain and accounts for nearly half of all exercise equipment sales in this country. In part, the popularity of the home exercise cycle is due to its simplicity, relative cheapness and ease of use, as well as to the fact that exercise cycles don't take up much space and are easily moved around the home. However, equally important is the fact that cycling does offer quite dramatic fitness benefits. The heart size and cardio-respiratory efficiency of top-class cyclists rivals that of the fittest distance runners and cross-country skiers. Cycling is also excellent for conditioning the muscles of the buttocks, hips, thighs and legs in general. The skill level associated with stationary cycling is also quite low, which makes it suitable for everybody, and since there is no foot strike, impact injuries are non-existent. This makes cycling, like walking, a very useful method of aerobic conditioning for the overweight, as well as for expectant mothers. Many athletes and sportsmen will also testify to the efficacy of cycling when it comes to maintaining fitness following injury, and in rehabilitation. A beginner's cycling programme is outlined in *Fig 25*.

BEGINNER'S CYCLING PROGRAMME

To begin with, start with little or no resistance, aiming for a smooth cycling rhythm of approximately 70 crank revolutions per minute. To work this out, count the number of times one foot pushes down: this will give you the crank revolution speed. Check your heart rate once you have been cycling easily at this rhythm. Once again, you are looking for a light to moderate exercise intensity. In terms of heart rate, you should be exercising at approximately 60 per cent of your predicted maximum. If you are not, increase the resistance slightly until this relative intensity has been reached.

Occasionally, check your exercise intensity as you cycle, and certainly do so as the weeks progress. As you become fitter, you may find that you have to increase the resistance setting to keep yourself working at 60 per cent MHR.

Working at this intensity, increase the time spent exercising according to the programme given here. As ever, remember to warm up and warm down thoroughly.

Once you can cycle easily every other day for at least 20 minutes, you can then start to make your cycling more demanding. This can be done in several ways. Naturally, increasing the resistance will make cycling harder, as will increasing the speed of cycling. By increasing the resistance for a short period of time, then going back to a lower resistance, or by increasing the speed and then slowing down, you can effectively mimic hills, do interval training and even perform fartlek cycling. How you cycle, once you are reasonably fit largely depends upon why you are training, as indicated at the beginning of this chapter.

Fig 25

Activity:	Cycling			
Week 1	Intensity	Duration (mins)	Resistance setting	Pedal/stroke frequency
Day 1	Aim for 60%	10	Suitable to	70 crank
Day 3	MHR in all	10	keep heart	revolutions
Day 5	sessions	10	rate at	per minute
Day 7		10	appropriate	
Week 2			value	
Day 2		10		
Day 4		12		
Day 6		10		
Week 3				
Day 1		10		
Day 3		12		
Day 5		10		
Day 7		12		
Week 4				
Day 2		10		
Day 4		15		
Day 6		10		
Week 5				
Day 1		12		
Day 3		10		
Day 5		15		
Day 7		10		
Week 6				
Day 2		15		
Day 4		15		
Day 6		15		

Fig 25

Week 7	Intensity	Duration (mins)	Resistance setting	Pedal/stroke frequency
Day 1		12		
Day 3		15		
Day 5		12		
Day 7		17		
Week 8				
Day 2		15		
Day 4		17		
Day 6		15		
Week 9				
Day 1		15		
Day 3		17		
Day 5		15		
Day 7		20		
Week 10				
Day 2		15		
Day 4		20		
Day 6		20		
Week 11				
Day 1		20		
Day 3		20		
Day 5		20		
Day 7		20		
Week 12				
Day 2		20		
Day 4		25		
Day 6		20		

Fig 25

Indoor cycling is also very popular since, like treadmill running, the weather is not a problem, and you do not have to contend with exhaust fumes and traffic. Regular home cyclists will also point to the fact that it is possible to do other things as you pedal along, including reading a book, listening to music and watching television. Potential drawbacks include the lack of changing scenery and cooling breeze, yet having said that, for ease of use and overall fitness benefits, a good quality exercise cycle is probably the best piece of home exercise equipment you can buy (*Fig 26*).

There are literally hundreds of different models to choose from when it comes to exercise cycles, of various qualities and in varying price brackets. If you are considering purchasing an exercise cycle the following essential buying tips should be borne in mind.

(a) Is it well-made? For regular and continuous use, with the minimum of maintenance, look for a model which is well-constructed with heavy gauge steel making up the frame. Remember, the more nuts and bolts a cycle has, the more parts there are to work loose.

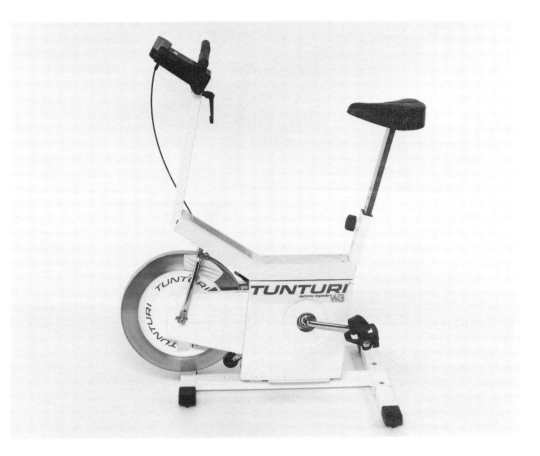

Fig 26 A typical home exercise cycle.

(b) Is it fully adjustable? For comfort and safety you should be able to adjust the height and position of both seat and handlebars. Saddle height is crucial. It should be possible to safely extend the saddle so that when seated your leg is almost fully extended when the pedal is in its lowest position. Check this, bearing in mind who else in your family may be using it, and note whether you have passed the safety limit indicated on the saddle post. Many of the cheaper models are not made for anyone much over 6ft tall. Likewise with the handlebars. Make sure that you can get into a comfortable cycling position without undue back or shoulder strain.

(c) Take a look at the flywheel and braking mechanism if possible. Generally speaking, the larger and heavier the flywheel, the smoother and more uniform the cycling action itself. There are various ways of braking the wheel to provide the resistance. Most commonly the resistance to pedalling is afforded by brake pads acting on the rim of the flywheel itself, or by a friction band around the wheel. Other methods involve air, and magnetic braking. Brake pad and friction systems are the easiest to maintain.

(d) A good cycle needs to have a number of instruments providing feedback about what you are doing. The resistance you are overcoming should certainly be indicated, be easily adjustable from light to very hard and all stages in between, and should be visible from the cycling position. There also needs to be some indication of just how fast you are going, and a readout of total distance covered. At times is also useful.

(e) Is the cycle comfortable and stable? There is only one way to check this, and that's to try it out for several minutes at varying speeds and resistances.

(f) Finally, does it fit the space you have in mind? Cycles vary in size and weight and in their manoeuvrability. Check this.

4. Rowing

After the exercise cycle, the next most popular single item of equipment for the home is a rowing machine. Rowing is another great general aerobic activity which is suitable for all types of people. Like cycling, it does not involve the impact of foot upon floor and is therefore suitable for the overweight, and anyone who is susceptible to impact induced injuries. Rowing also has an added advantage in that it conditions the muscles of the upper body as well as those of the legs, making it a good overall exercise activity to choose. However, rowing is not a suitable activity for individuals with certain back problems, although paradoxically it may help cure some back conditions. If you do have any back trouble, check the suitability of rowing as a form of exercise with your GP first.

A beginner's rowing programme is outlined in *Fig 27*.

BEGINNER'S ROWING PROGRAMME

As with cycling, begin with little or no resistance, aiming for a stroke frequency of approximately 16 – 20 strokes per minute. Check your heart rate after a couple of minutes. Increase the resistance according to the manufacturers' instructions so that your heart rate is approximately 60 per cent of maximum, if necessary. As you progress through the programme, keep a check on your heart rate and adjust the resistance of your machine so that your heart rate is always at the appropriate level.

Remember to warm up and warm down thoroughly.

For guidelines for advanced rowers see cycling programme (Page 48).

Fig 27

Activity:	Rowing			
Week 1	Intensity	Duration (mins)	Resistance setting	Pedal/stroke frequency
Day 1	Aim for 60%	5	Suitable to	16 – 20
Day 3	MHR in all	5	keep heart	strokes per
Day 5	sessions	5	rate at	minute
Day 7		5	appropriate	
			value	
Week 2				
Day 2		5		
Day 4		7		
Day 6		5		
Week 3				
Day 1		5		
Day 3		7		
Day 5		5		
Day 7		7		
Week 4				
Day 2		5		
Day 4		10		
Day 6		5		
Week 5				
Day 1		5		
Day 3		7		
Day 5		5		
Day 7		10		
Week 6				
Day 2		7		
Day 4		10		
Day 6		7		

Fig 27

Week 7	Intensity	Duration (mins)	Resistance setting	Pedal/stroke frequency
Day 1		7		
Day 3		10		
Day 5		7		
Day 7		10		
Week 8				
Day 2		10		
Day 4		10		
Day 6		10		
Week 9				
Day 1		10		
Day 3		12		
Day 5		10		
Day 7		12		
Week 10				
Day 2		12		
Day 4		12		
Day 6		12		
Week 11				
Day 1		10		
Day 3		12		
Day 5		10		
Day 7		15		
Week 12				
Day 2		15		
Day 4		15		
Day 6		15		

Fig 27

Whilst there are numerous rowers on the market, it is possible to group the various models into one of two categories: those which rely on hydraulic cylinders to provide the resistance, and those which do not. The first type are the most inexpensive and the type you are most likely to find in sports stores (*Fig 28*). Basically, hydraulic machines have hydraulic cylinders to which the rowing handles ('oars') are attached. The cylinders invariably have some method of increasing the resistance to make the rowing action more or less demanding. (If the machine you are thinking of purchasing does not feature a method of varying the resistance, it is really not worth buying, since you will be unable to progress or structure interesting exercise programmes). As with an exercise cycle, it

should be possible to vary the resistance quickly from very easy to very hard. The sturdier and more robust the cylinders, the more positive the rowing action. Check, too, that the two cylinders afford the same resistance and that the action is smooth and quiet. The only real way to do this is to try the machine out. This will also let you see whether you can go through a full range of movement. A good rower will allow you to move from a position when your knees are close to your chest, to a position where your legs are fully extended.

Since you will be spending some time on it, the seat should feel comfortable and slide easily along its rollers or track. The seat on a well-made machine will be contoured to fit your behind, and will slide effortlessly in near

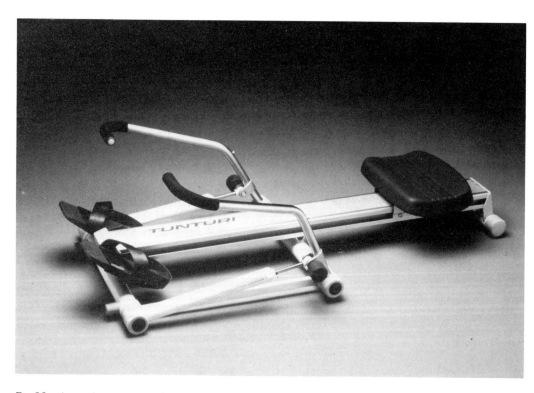

Fig 28   A simple rowing machine.

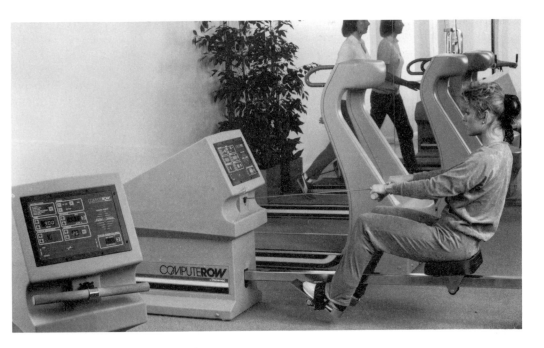

Fig 29   A computerised rowing machine.

silence. Good rowers also have footplates and straps to anchor your feet in position.

As with all exercise machines, your chosen rower needs to offer feedback about the exercise you are doing. Useful displays are those which show resistance, stroke rate, and time spent exercising. Finally, check that it fits into the space that you have in mind.

The other types of rowing machine that you are likely to see advertised are more substantial than the hydraulic rowers described, and actually feel more like rowing on water (*Fig 29*). These machines are often referred to as 'straight-pull' rowers, and have only one handle, with the resistance being offered by an electromagnetic or air braking system. They are considerably more expensive than hydraulic models. They also tend to be very long (some versions being 2.5m in length) and somewhat noisier than other rowing machines, too. A number of straight-pull

models also have built-in video display units and LED consoles which allow you to programme the machine so that you can 'race' against another rower who appears on the display panel, either as a moving light or as a miniature man-in-a-boat. Some electronic versions even reproduce the sound of oars cutting through the water as you row, as well as offering applause when you beat your opponent to the finish line.

As with the electronic cycles which have similar feedback gadgets, you will pay a considerable amount of money for all these extras. The training effect is no different from similar machines without the gadgets, but you may find that such high-tech machines offer a great deal of motivation, as well as being good fun. If you are not a committed exerciser, such machines, whilst being expensive, may persuade you to exercise on a more regular basis.

Structurally, a straight-pull machine should be robust and well made. Again, try before you buy, checking ease of use, range of movement, work-out information displays and operational space requirements.

Good rowing technique is a must if you are to get the most from your rower and avoid injury. The sequence of diagrams in *Fig 30* shows how to row correctly. To begin the drive (a), the rower reaches forward with knees bent, arms extended, and body leaning toward the flywheel. The drive is begun with the legs and the back doing all the work. Note that the arms are straight and the shoulders relaxed.

Halfway through the drive (b), the legs and back are still doing all the work. The arms are still straight with the shoulders still relaxed. At the finish of the drive (c), the handle is pulled by the arms and shoulders into the abdomen. The legs are straight and the body is leaning back slightly. Note that the height of the handle is neither at the chest nor in the lap.

The first motion of the recovery (d) is to extend the arms and swing the body forward at the hips. This puts the handle in front of the knees to avoid interference between the knees and hands as the seat moves forward.

The body is drawn forward with the legs to the starting position (e) for the next stroke. The rower is now ready to begin the next drive. Remember that your body should never come to a complete stop.

Most people find rowing quite demanding. You may like to keep progressing in the manner described until you are exercising for longer, according to your training aim, or, as with cycling, adjusting the stroke frequency and/or the resistance enables you to interval train or mimic hard going 'on the water'.

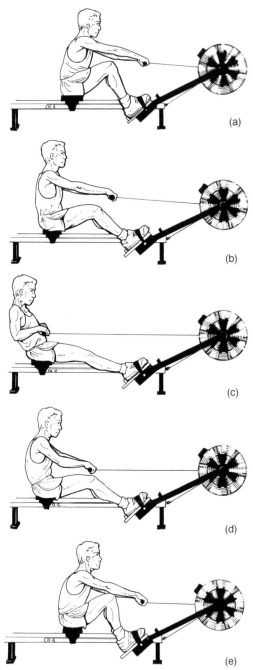

(a)

(b)

(c)

(d)

(e)

Fig 30 The correct indoor rowing technique for the Concept II Rowing Ergometer.

5. Stair and Climbing Machines

In the last few years quite a number of new machines have been developed with the home exercise market in mind. Many of these new items of exercise equipment rely upon some form of stepping or climbing action, with some even featuring what looks like a small set of continuously revolving stairs. All the stair or stepping machines use your body weight as resistance and allow you to work at different speeds or stepping rates, with some versions offering you the option of having a shorter or longer stride (*Fig 31*). As with many items of home exercise equipment, the most expensive models feature all kinds of video displays of workload and general exercise information, with some having built-in fitness tests and programable options allowing for interval training, for example.

Stair climbing or continuous stepping can be excellent aerobic exercise and is a very good conditioning exercise for the muscles of the lower body, particularly the muscles of the buttocks. It is suitable for most people and has a very low injury risk. The major drawback as far as most people are concerned is the fact that stair climbing or continuous stepping is extremely boring, although the screen and programmes of the expensive, computerised machines do make these forms of exercise more interesting.

Other machines in a similar vein also aim to condition the muscles of the upper body, as well as those of the lower half, by providing a climbing option through handles which move as you step up and down (*Fig 32*). The rate of climbing and the resistance and range of movement can all be varied on the best models. These machines are excellent for general muscle conditioning as well as for improving aerobic fitness. However, they are still very expensive and can also be quite monotonous. The other potential drawback of

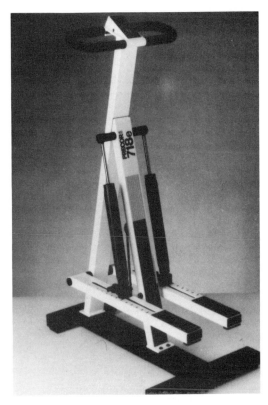

Fig 31   Home 'stepping' unit.

such climbing machines is that they need a lot of vertical space, often being around 2.5m high.

All stair, stepping and climbing machines need to be robust, smooth and quiet in operation. They should allow you to exercise at varying intensities and should provide clear information about the workload of your exercise session. Certainly you need to know the resistance you are overcoming and your stepping or climbing rate, as well as the time spent exercising.

Because of the diverse nature of such products it is difficult to give a definite training programme. The principles of training and structuring the programme are, however,

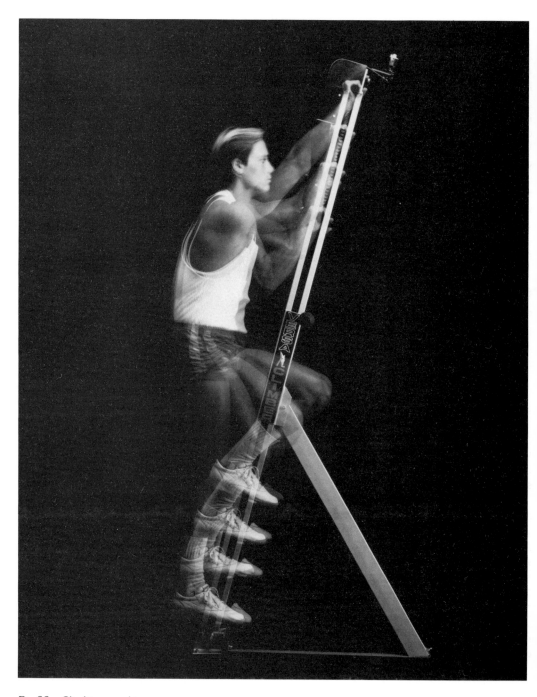

Fig 32   Climbing machine.

identical to any of the other pieces of exercise equipment given here. Use your heart rate as an indicator of exercise intensity as outlined earlier, and aim to exercise continuously for as long as is comfortable, every other day. Try and extend the total time spent exercising as the weeks go by until you are exercising continuously for approximately 20 minutes. When you can do this, you can then introduce exercise at higher resistances or at higher stepping or climbing frequencies. Record your training in your training log. Fortunately, all stair, stepping and climbing machines come with clear instructions on how the training load can be varied and progressed according to fitness.

6. Skiing Machines

The last few years have also seen the introduction of skiing machines for home exercise. These pieces of exercise equipment are designed so that you can mimic the action of cross-country skiing, which is generally regarded as an excellent overall conditioning activity (*Fig 33*). Again, there are a number of different versions of skiing machines, but they all have a similar design. All have footplates which can glide along runners. These should move easily and allow you to take longer or shorter strides according to fitness.

There should also be some method of increasing or decreasing the resistance acting upon the footplates so that the exercise can be made progressively more demanding. All skiing machines also feature some form of upper body resistance acting as the 'poles'. Again the resistance and range of movement of this part of the machine should be variable. There should be visual information about resistance and workload being overcome clearly displayed on the machine.

Again, designs vary, and it's best to try before you buy, looking for robustness, ease of use and space requirements. Exact training details will vary according to the model you may choose, but the principles outlined for stair and stepping machines should be followed.

OTHER AEROBIC FITNESS OPTIONS

Other options are available for improving aerobic fitness in the home, yet they tend not to be as effective as those activities mentioned already. One such option is 'Rebounding'. This activity is carried out on what looks like a miniature trampoline, called a Rebounder. Basically you can run, jump and hop on the Rebounder, as well as being able to carry out other simple exercises. Proponents of the Rebounding system argue that it is the most effective method of improving aerobic fitness, but there is no documented research to substantiate such claims. In fact, independent research studies have shown that Rebounding is a poor method of improving aerobic fitness in the averagely fit person. The best use of the Rebounder is in rehabilitation from injury, or as a form of exercise for the very unfit and overweight.

Skipping is also put forward as a viable method of improving aerobic fitness. Yet whilst skipping is inexpensive, a high skill level is needed and most people will find that they cannot skip continuously for long enough to gain an aerobic training effect. Skipping is also not recommended for the overweight and unfit.

Finally, there are many exercise videos available which feature aerobic exercise phases. Perhaps their biggest drawback is the fact that once you can do the exercises given in the video you can no longer progress and improve fitness. Some videos also feature poor exercise programmes. If you are going to purchase a video to exercise to, make sure it has been put together by a qualified instructor.

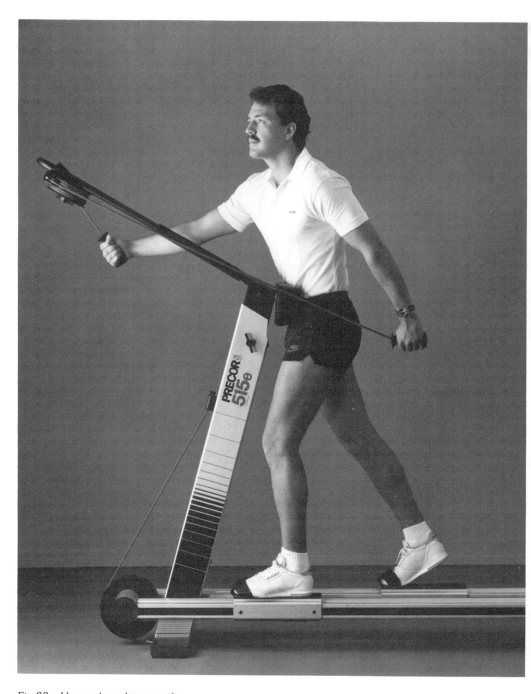

Fig 33   Heavy-duty skiing machine.

The chart in *Fig 34* summarises the different aerobic fitness options.

Activity	Benefits	Disadvantages	Cost	Space needed	Body part bias
Walking	Easy. Requires little equipment. Suitable for all age groups and the very unfit.	Not demanding enough for the fitter person to improve overall fitness.	Very cheap	Outdoors	Lower body
Jogging/running	Easy. Little equipment needed.	May pose injury problems for the overweight.	Cheap	Outdoors	Lower body

(Note: if the above activities are carried out on a treadmill, they become expensive and require floor space of approximately 2m × 1m.)

Activity	Benefits	Disadvantages	Cost	Space needed	Body part bias
Cycling	Easy. Suitable for all age groups and fitness levels.	Can be boring. Some cycles are very noisy	Cheap to expensive – depends on model	1m²	Lower body
Rowing	Easy. Works all major muscle groups.	Not suitable for the unfit or those with back problems.	Cheap to expensive – depends on model	2m × 1m	
Stair machines	Everyday activity.	Very boring	Very expensive	1.5m²	Lower body
Climbing machines	All-body activity	Very boring.	Very expensive	floor space 1m²	
Skiing machines	All-body activity	Unnatural action for many people.	Expensive	2m × 1m	
Rebounding	Easy. Suitable for the very unfit and those with joint problems.	Inadequate for real training.	Cheap	1m²	Lower body
Skipping	Little equipment needed.	High skill level needed.	Cheap	2m × 2m	Lower body

Fig 34   Summary of aerobic exercise activities.

6 Exercise for Muscular Strength and Endurance

Exercising with the aim of improving either muscular strength or muscular endurance involves asking your muscles to overcome some form of resistance. The resistance which muscles must overcome can be offered in a number of ways. Your own body weight can be used very effectively, as can some form of external weight, like barbells and dumb-bells. There are also numerous resistance machines available for the task featuring weight blocks, hydraulic cylinders, electromagnetic braking, springs and rubber bands.

If exercising with a view to improving muscular strength, the resistance you overcome must be high. To give an example, if you were using a barbell, you would choose a weight which would allow you to carry out a given exercise perhaps as few as six times. This set of six repetitions of an exercise would then be repeated, after a short recovery, four or five times, before moving on to an exercise for another muscle group. In terms of the maximum resistance (weight) you could overcome in an exercise, strength training requires you to work at around 85 per cent of your maximum. Muscular endurance training, on the other hand, does not require you to work so intensely. A typical muscular endurance schedule, for example, would require you to complete an exercise with a barbell at least fifteen times. This set of fifteen

repetitions would then be repeated after a short recovery perhaps three times, before moving on to another exercise, although, as with strength training, there are variations on this basic theme as indicated later on in this chapter. (*Figs 35–39*.) In terms of maximum resistance, endurance programmes require you to work at approximately 50–60 per cent of your maximum.

Obviously, varying the resistance and consequently the number of times you perform an exercise, makes it possible to use the same exercise for either improving strength, or improving endurance. All you really need to bear in mind is that strength training programmes require high resistances and low repetitions, whilst endurance programmes require low resistances and high repetitions.

Strength training programmes are very demanding, and do place considerable stresses upon muscles and joints. Because of this, it is best to spend several weeks working through a general muscular endurance programme, as given in this chapter, (*Fig 35*) before carrying out a strength-training regime as in *Fig 40*. An aerobic fitness activity, plus flexibility exercises, should also accompany endurance or strength-training programmes if you are to achieve total fitness.

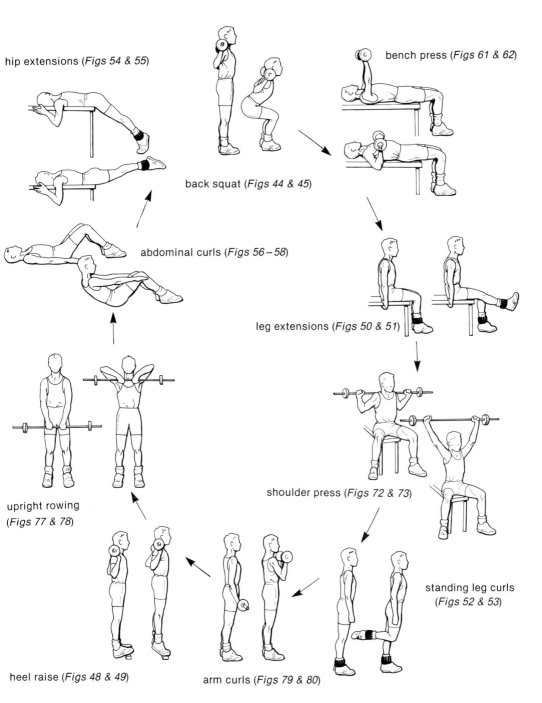

hip extensions (*Figs 54 & 55*)

back squat (*Figs 44 & 45*)

bench press (*Figs 61 & 62*)

abdominal curls (*Figs 56 – 58*)

leg extensions (*Figs 50 & 51*)

upright rowing
(*Figs 77 & 78*)

shoulder press (*Figs 72 & 73*)

standing leg curls
(*Figs 52 & 53*)

heel raise (*Figs 48 & 49*)

arm curls (*Figs 79 & 80*)

Fig 35   Sample beginner's general endurance programme.

SAMPLE BEGINNER'S GENERAL ENDURANCE PROGRAMME

Back squat	*(Figs 45 & 46)*
Bench press	*(Figs 62 & 63)*
Leg extensions	*(Figs 51 & 52)*
Shoulder press	*(Figs 72 & 73)*
Standing leg curls	*(Figs 53 & 54)*
Arm curls	*(Figs 79 & 80)*
Heel raise	*(Figs 49 & 50)*
Upright rowing	*(Figs 77 & 78)*
Abdominal curls	*(Figs 57 – 59)*
Hip extensions	*(Figs 55 & 56)*

This muscular endurance programme can be made more aerobic. Carry out the programme in the above sequence yet, instead of moving straight on to the next exercise, introduce one minute of low intensity aerobic activity between exercises. The activity chosen can be any of those given in Chapter 5, and will depend upon the availability of equipment and where you are exercising. An example of a combined aerobic/muscular endurance programme is given in *Fig 39*, using cycling as the aerobic activity.

Fig 35

Resistance exercises can also be used in conjunction with an aerobic activity to produce a number of general training benefits. Basically, after a warm-up, a resistance exercise is performed, followed by aerobic activity, followed by a resistance exercise, etc. This sequence of aerobic activity followed by resistance exercise is known as aerobic circuit weight training and is a very useful and effective training method if time is short, and can easily be performed in the home setting with simple equipment. (A typical programme is given in *Fig 39*.) Strength and endurance programmes can also be structured to work on certain parts of the body. Again, sample programmes are given in *Figs 36–38*. *Fig 40* shows a general strength programme. For best results, exercise every other day.

SAMPLE BEGINNER'S UPPER BODY PROGRAMME

Bench press	*(Figs 62 & 63)*
Dumb-bell flyes	*(Figs 70 & 71)*
Shoulder press	*(Figs 72 & 73)*
Lateral raise	*(Fig 76)*
Arm curls	*(Figs 79 & 80)*
Upright rowing	*(Figs 77 & 78)*
Abdominal crunch	*(Figs 60 & 61)*
Hip extensions	*(Figs 55 & 56)*

Figs 36 – 38   Specific body part endurance programmes.

SAMPLE BEGINNER'S LOWER BODY PROGRAMME

Back squat	*(Figs 45 & 46)*
Bench stepping	*(Figs 47 & 48)*
Leg extension	*(Figs 51 & 52)*
Standing leg curls	*(Figs 53 & 54)*
Heel raise	*(Figs 49 & 50)*
Hip extensions	*(Figs 55 & 56)*

Fig 37

SAMPLE BEGINNER'S BODY PART PROGRAMME: ABDOMINALS

Abdominal curls	*(Figs 57 – 59)*
Abdominal crunch	*(Figs 60 & 61)*
Abdominal curls (diagonal)	*(Fig 59)*

This sequence to be repeated four times, with a recovery period of 1 minute between circuits.

Fig 38

SAMPLE BEGINNER'S AEROBIC/MUSCULAR ENDURANCE PROGRAMME

Back squat 1 minute easy cycling	*(Figs 45 & 46)*
Bench press 1 minute easy cycling	*(Figs 62 & 63)*
Leg extensions 1 minute easy cycling	*(Figs 51 & 52)*
Shoulder press 1 minute easy cycling	*(Figs 72 & 73)*
Standing leg curls 1 minute easy cycling	*(Figs 53 & 54)*
Arm curls 1 minute easy cycling	*(Figs 79 & 80)*
Heel raise 1 minute easy cycling	*(Figs 49 & 50)*
Upright rowing 1 minute easy cycling	*(Figs 77 & 78)*
Abdominal curls 1 minute easy cycling	*(Figs 79 & 80)*
Hip extensions 1 minute easy cycling	*(Figs 55 & 56)*

This programme is quite demanding. Keep the weights/resistances low to begin with. No resistance setting on your cycle, 70 crank revolutions per minute. 1 circuit initially.

Fig 39

SAMPLE BEGINNERS' GENERAL STRENGTH PROGRAMME
(Each exercise to be performed in four sets of six, with 90 seconds recovery between sets.)

Back squats	*(Figs 45 & 46)*
Bench press	*(Figs 62 & 63)*
Leg extensions	*(Figs 51 & 52)*
Shoulder press	*(Figs 72 & 73)*
Standing leg curls	*(Figs 53 & 54)*
Arm curls	*(Figs 79 & 80)*
Heel raise	*(Figs 49 & 50)*
Upright rowing	*(Figs 77 & 78)*
Abdominal curls	*(Figs 57 – 59)*
Hip extensions	*(Figs 55 & 56)*

The specific body part programmes given in the muscular endurance section (*Figs 35 to 37*) can be adapted in a similar way to emphasise strength rather than endurance.

Fig 40

EQUIPMENT

A number of resistance exercises are given in this chapter which involve only your own body weight and they can be used very effectively to achieve strength or endurance-training benefits. However, the purchase of simple equipment does make a wider range of exercise choices available, and may make some exercises more effective.

The most basic equipment to choose from is some form of strap-on ankle/wrist weight set. These come in a variety of weights and make arm and leg exercises more demanding. As indicated in the previous chapter, they may also be used to increase the intensity of walking (Power Walking). If purchasing such weights, make sure that they can be securely fastened around your limbs and are not likely to fly off during more vigorous movements. It is better to buy too light a set of ankle/wrist weights than too heavy a pair: 1kg is probably about right for most beginners.

After such strap-on weights, the next most basic purchase is some form of dumb-bell or barbell set. Dumb-bells and barbells come in all forms and weights. The cheapest versions are usually a heavy material, like concrete or sand, encased in vinyl or plastic. Such versions, whilst effective, do tend to be very bulky, lacking the density of a material like iron, the more common, if slightly more expensive material for weight sets. A very wide range of exercises can be performed with a simple dumb-bell or barbell kit, as indicated in the exercise section of this chapter. If purchasing a weights kit, bear in mind that you will need at least two dumb-bell rods, four collars (to secure the weights at each end) and an equal number of weight discs so that the ends of the dumb-bells, as well as the dumb-bells themselves, are balanced. A range of smaller discs is perhaps better than a few large discs, since you can increase the weights in more appropriate increments as you become

fitter. Remember that you can always buy loose discs to add to your dumb-bell or barbell set. Some dumb-bells are of a fixed weight and do not allow for the addition of discs at each end. If you are considering the purchase of such dumb-bells, bear in mind that you will have to have two of each in differing weights, which could be costly. The same is true of barbells. Barbell rods also come in different lengths. A relatively long bar (1.85m/6ft) may mean that you will have to have more exercise space, but it will mean that certain exercises can be carried out more comfortably, most notably the squat. Again, choose a range of smaller discs rather than a few large ones.

Other than the purchase of the weights themselves, you may consider buying a bench and stands so that you can add more exercises to your schedule for variety. The stronger, more stable and more robust this type of equipment, the better. Benches and stands should preferably be manufactured from steel box section of large diameter (40mm minimum) and should have few bolt-on sections. Good quality benches also have an adjustable seat so that still more exercises can be performed. Stands should also have a heavy base so that they do not fall over easily.

Some manufacturers have also produced benches which have additional features, like leg curl/extension attachments. Only extremely well-made benches can handle the extra stresses placed upon them during such exercises and allow you to carry out the exercise safely and effectively (*Fig 41*). Try out any such attachment if you are considering the purchase of this type of bench, and note whether the attachment moves, squeaks or wobbles as you do the exercise. If it does not feel secure and functional, do not bother.

Moving on from dumb-bells and barbells, the next option in home resistance equipment is some form of multi-gym. These devices are designed so that you can perform a number of

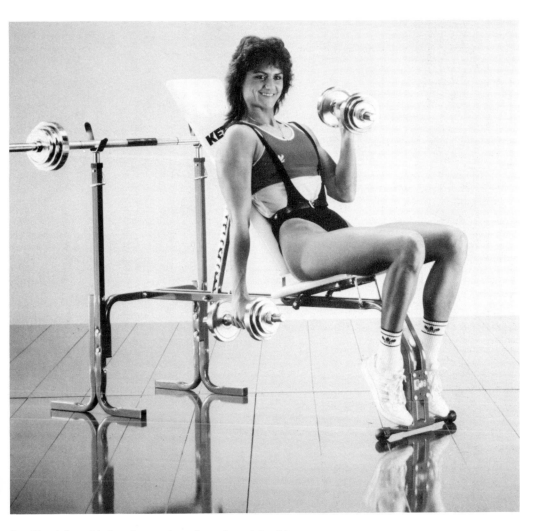

Fig 41   Adjustable bench, stands and weight-training kit..

different exercises, often using just one centrally placed weight stack. Through a series of cables and pulleys, the weights are moved up and down a pair of runners. There are few good cheap multi-gyms for home use available (*Fig 42*). Many of the inexpensive models have small weight stacks (making many exercises ineffective after a period of a few weeks of training). Further, the weights do not move easily along the runners, pulleys are often off-centre and the general quality of materials used is poor. And, whilst the manufacturers make claims for an unbelievable number of exercises which the equipment can accommodate, very often the execution of many of the exercises requires a virtual rebuilding of the machine. Such items also take up considerable floor space.

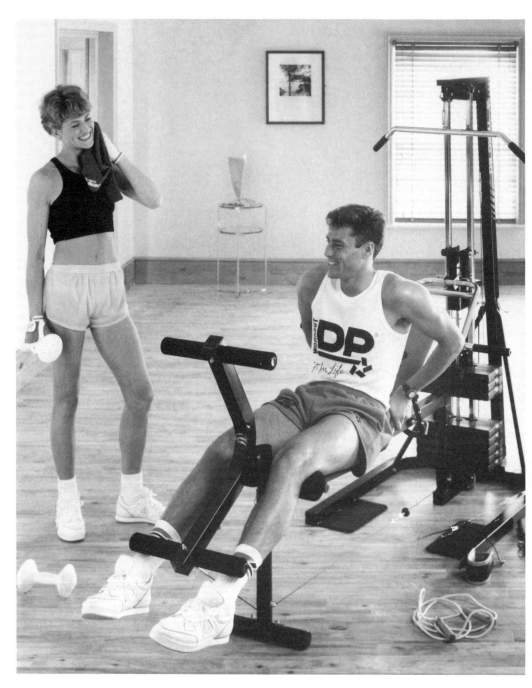

Fig 42   *A typical home multi-exercise unit.*

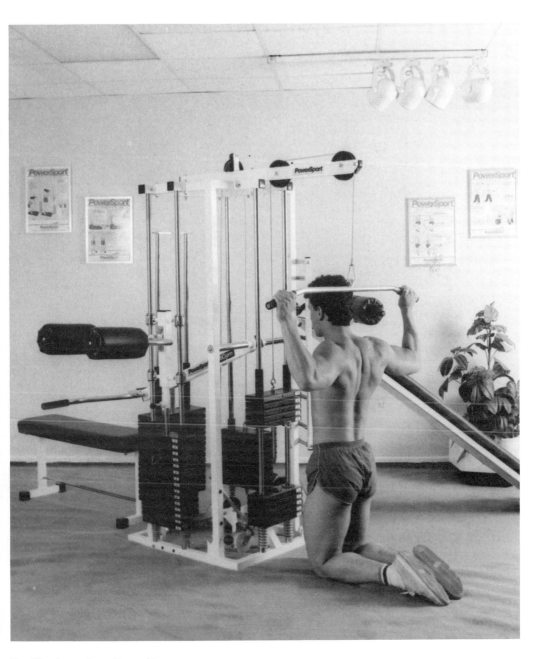

Fig 43   A good quality multi-gym.

Equipment	Benefits	Disadvantages	Cost	Space needed
Ankle/wrist weights	Allow for the execution of many extra exercises.	Too light for certain strength training-exercises.	Cheap	2m × 1m
Dumb-bells	Allow for execution of many more exercises and more serious strength training.	Do not allow you to carry out certain exercises involving two hands. Amount of weight limited.	Cheap	2m × 1m
Barbell kit	Allows you to carry out a large number of strength-training exercises.	Starts to take up more space and starts to cost more money. Some exercises may need help of a partner.	Moderately expensive	2.5m × 1.5m
Bench/stands	Allow you to do certain barbell exercises more safely. Essential for serious strength training.	Takes up even more space.	Moderately expensive	2.5m × 2m (including weights)
Multi-gym	Full range of exercises which can be done safely on your own.	Takes up a great deal of space. Good ones are expensive.	Expensive	2.5m × 2.5m (average)

Fig 44   Resistance training equipment summary.

More expensive models are good, however. These are often merely scaled down versions of the multi-gym equipment you would find in a health club and function in a similar way (*Fig 43*). They also take up a considerable amount of space, but if you have this, and the money, they are a good option for the whole family.

Some multi-gym models work not through weights, but by having a series of hydraulic cylinders incorporated in their design. This makes them much lighter and far more movable than traditional weight-based machines, and they are often smaller. You do have to pay more for these features, however.

If shopping with home resistance training equipment in mind, you will find promotional material from each manufacturer explaining why their equipment is better than anyone else's. To be honest, it doesn't really matter how you overcome the resistance or what type of resistance you overcome as far as general fitness is concerned. You should be more concerned about good quality construction, machines which allow a full range of movement whatever your size, are easy to use and are comfortable. The only way to know this, once again, is to road-test any potential purchase thoroughly. This means trying out every exercise you are supposed to be able to do on it, and comparing it to other machines. If it feels good, fits your space and your budget and you think you'll use it on a regular basis, buy it.

Fig 44 gives a summary of the relative benefits of resistance training equipment.

RESISTANCE EXERCISES

This section lists a number of common exercises which feature in the various exercise programmes given in this book. They use body weight, or simple equipment only and give an idea of the variety of exercises you can do. A more extensive range of resistance exercises is given in the companion book *The Complete Book of Resistance Training*.

Follow all exercise instructions as carefully as possible, repeating the exercise as often as is required according to the exercise programme you are following. The following safety rules should also be borne in mind when using resistance training equipment:

Warm up thoroughly.

Exercise from a stable base.

Wear suitable shoes.

Lift and lower weights to the floor with a straight back, bending at the knees.

Only add or remove weights from a bar when it is safely on the floor.

Always check any equipment you are about to use for safety, including collar tightness.

Get the help of a partner for awkward free weight exercises.

Adjust any other equipment according to manufacturers' recommendations.

Maintain control of any weights you are using at all times, performing each exercise smoothly, without forcing or jerking.

Warm down thoroughly.

In addition, never sacrifice exercise technique just to lift heavier weights or to perform more repetitions of an exercise.

The following muscular endurance programmes should be performed using a weight/exercise position sufficiently heavy/intense so that you can just manage fifteen repetitions of each exercise: this will require trial and error initially. Aim for good technique throughout all the exercises and move swiftly from one exercise to another. Complete one circuit of the exercises to begin with. As you become fitter, increase the number of times you do the circuit, aiming eventually to perform 3 complete circuits, one after the other. When this is easy, increase the weights, or make the exercise position more demanding (as indicated in the exercise instructions) on some or all of the exercises, still aiming to complete fifteen repetitions of each exercise. Remember to warm up and warm down thoroughly as part of your total exercise session.

Naturally, the exercise programmes given here are samples only. Depending upon the equipment you have, you may be able to choose many more exercises with which to structure your programmes.

For best results, exercise every other day.

1. Back Squat
(*Figs 45 & 46*)

This is the most useful conditioning exercise for the muscles of the legs, back and buttocks, and forms the core of many training programmes. Stand tall with you feet approximately shoulder-width apart. Rest a barbell comfortably across your shoulders/upper back. (Squat stands will certainly make it easier to position the weight accurately). Keep your spine long, look forward and bend your knees, squatting under control to a position where your thighs are parallel to the floor. Hold this position momentarily, then smoothly return to your starting position, straightening your legs fully. Breathe in as you descend, and out as you rise. If, whilst you are doing the exercise, you find that your heels leave the floor, place a block of wood (approximately 2.5cm high) under your heels. This exercise can also be done holding a dumb-bell in each hand, as illustrated.

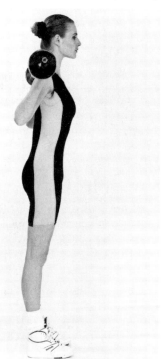
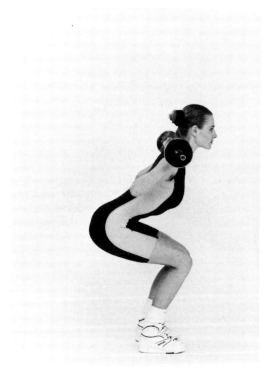

Figs 45 and 46   Back squat.

2. Bench Stepping (*Fig 47 & 48*)

This warming-up exercise described in Chapter 4 can also be used with more resistance to condition the legs, thighs and buttocks. Rest a barbell across the shoulders/ upper back, as in the previous exercise, and step up and down on the bench, as outlined on page 28. Dumb-bells held in either hand will also achieve the same conditioning effect. Start with a light weight to begin with, since you will need to acquire a certain amount of balance initially.

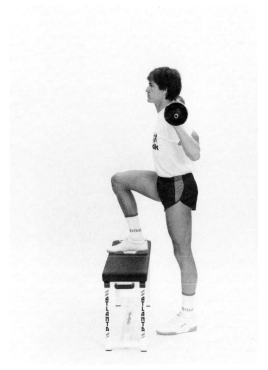
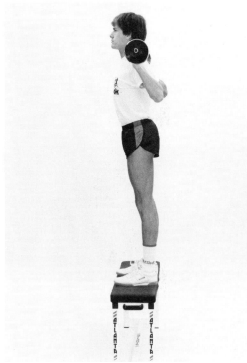

Figs 47 and 48   Bench stepping.

3. Heel Raise
(*Figs 49 & 50*)

This is a great exercise for the calf muscles. Stand tall with a barbell resting across your upper back/shoulders, or have two dumbbells in your hands. Rest the balls of your feet on a block of wood (approximately 2.5cm high) and keep your heels on the floor. Keeping your spine long and looking straight ahead, rise up on to your toes. Hold your uppermost position momentarily, then control the movement of your heels back towards the floor. As soon as your heels touch the ground, smoothly repeat the sequence. Breathe normally throughout the exercise.

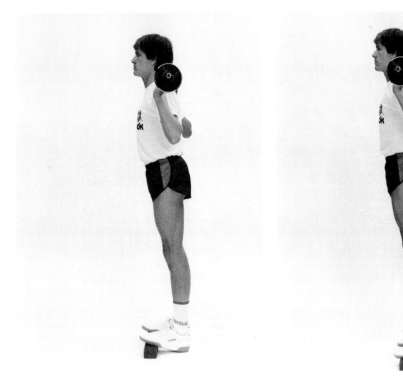

Figs 49 and 50   Heel raise.

4. Leg Extensions (*Figs 51 & 52*)

This exercise is excellent for conditioning the muscles at the front of the thigh. You will need ankle weights strapped to both legs. Sit on the edge of a bench or table so that your knees are just off its edge. Hold on to the sides of the bench and keep your spine long. From this position, smoothly straighten your legs, and hold their fully straightened position momentarily before lowering them under control back to the starting position, and repeat. Breathe normally throughout the sequence.

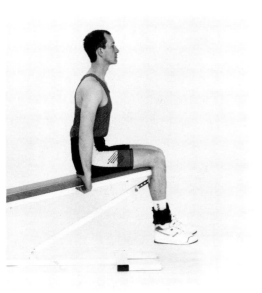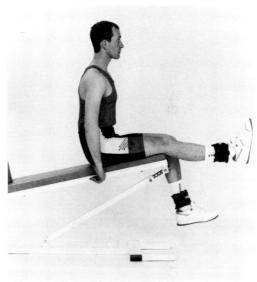

Figs 51 and 52   Leg extensions.

5. Standing Leg Curls (*Figs 53 & 54*)

This exercise conditions the muscles of the back of the thigh. Stand tall, wearing your ankle weights, using a chair-back or something similar for support. Keeping your pelvis centred and in the same place throughout the exercise, smoothly raise one heel towards your buttocks, supporting your weight on the other leg. Hold your uppermost position momentarily, then lower your leg, under control, back to the starting position. Repeat the appropriate number of times, then perform the exercise on the other leg. Breathe normally throughout.

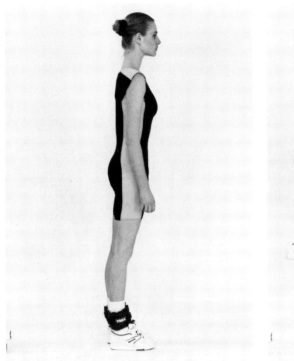
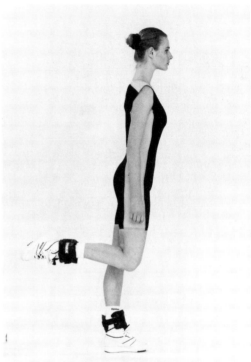

Figs 53 and 54   Standing leg curls.

6. Hip Extensions (*Figs 55 & 56*)

This is a very good exercise for conditioning the muscles of the buttocks, lower back and backs of legs in general. Lie face down on a long table, firmly gripping its sides and pressing your hips firmly against it. Your feet should be resting on the floor. Keeping your legs straight, slowly raise them towards the ceiling. When they are parallel to the floor, hold this position momentarily, then lower them smoothly to the starting position. As your feet touch the floor, repeat. Breathe in as you raise your legs, and out as you lower them. This exercise can be made progressively harder by adding weights to your ankles.

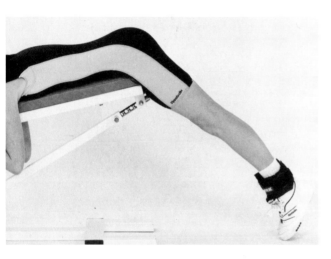

Figs 55 and 56   Hip extensions.

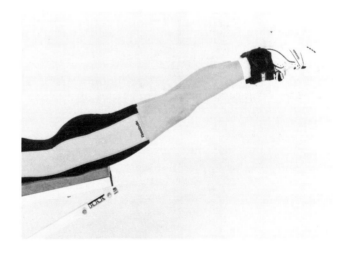

7. Abdominal Curls (*Figs 57 – 59*)

This is the key exercise for conditioning the muscles at the front of the trunk. Lie flat on the floor, with your knees bent at an angle of approximately 90 degrees. Rest your arms, folded, across your chest, or have them loosely by your sides, making sure that your lower back is pressed strongly into the floor at all times; smoothly curl your head and shoulders off the floor aiming to touch your thighs with your arms. The fitter you become, the closer to your thighs you will be able to go.

Having reached your uppermost position, slowly curl down, and repeat as soon as your mid-back touches the floor. Breathe out as you curl up, and breathe in as you curl down. This exercise can be made progressively harder by moving your hands to a position where your fingertips are resting loosely by the side of your head.

A variation of this exercise (*Fig 59*) is to twist to the side as you curl up: this makes the side abdominal muscles work harder. The twist should begin as you being the curl up. Twist equally to both sides.

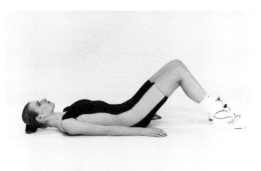
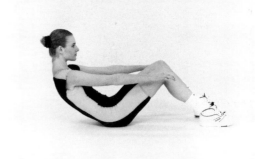

Figs 57 & 58   Abdominal curl.

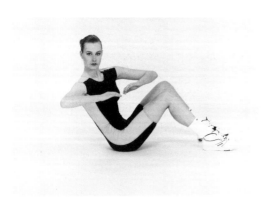

Fig 59   Twisting Abdominal curl.

8. Abdominal Crunch (*Figs 60 & 61*)

This is another good abdominal exercise. Lie flat on the floor, with your legs above you so that your knees are directly over your abdomen. Now try and perform the curl up as before, but hold your uppermost position momentarily before curling down. Curl down and repeat, breathing as before.

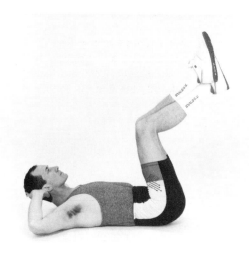

Figs 60 and 61   Abdominal crunch.

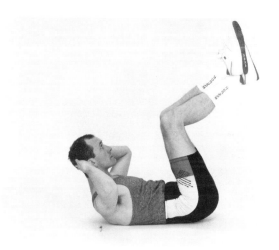

9. Bench Press (*Figs 62 & 63*)

This exercise is for the muscles of the chest predominantly, although it also conditions the muscles at the front of the shoulder, as well as those at the back of the upper arms. For the exercise you will need a barbell and bench, unless you have a multi-gym with a bench-pressing station. Lie with your back flat on the bench, making sure that your lower back is firmly pressed into it, holding the barbell at arm's length, with a wide grip, above your chest (use stands or a partner to help you get into the starting position). Steadily lower the bar so that it touches your chest, then press it smoothly upwards to arm's length again, and repeat. Breathe in as you lower the bar, and breathe out as you raise it.

(Note that in all pressing exercises like this, you should aim to keep your elbows under the bar and have a straight wrist so that all your effort is directed through the barbell).

If your bench has an inclined seat, raising the seat causes this exercise to work the muscles of the upper chest and shoulders more.

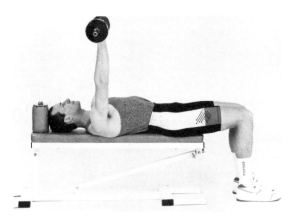

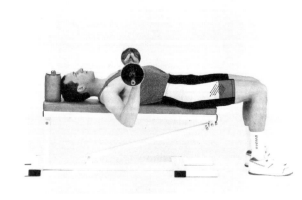

Figs 62 and 63   Bench press.

84

10. Press-ups
(Figs 64 – 69)

In the absence of any equipment, the press-up exercise conditions the same muscles as the bench press exercise. Done correctly, it also works the muscles of the trunk (*Fig 64*). Take a starting position, as illustrated. Note that your hands are underneath your shoulders and that there is effectively a straight line running from your ankles through your knees, hips and shoulders. Bend at your elbows so that your chest moves towards the floor. Go as far as you can, hold your position for a moment, then straighten your arms and repeat. Breathe in as you lower yourself towards the floor, and breathe out as you return to your starting position.

This exercise is quite demanding. It can be made easier by starting from a kneeling position, as shown, or easier still by starting more upright and performing the action against a wall. It can be made more difficult by starting the exercise with your feet up on a bench. Choose whichever exercise position is most appropriate for you according to your fitness level and training aim.

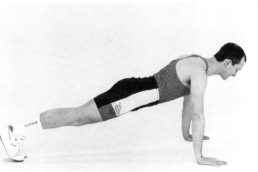 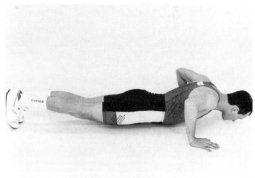

Figs 64 and 65   Press-ups.

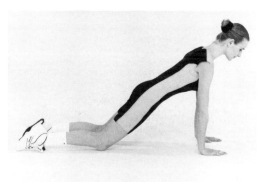 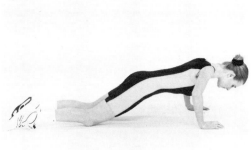

Figs 66 and 67   Knee press-ups.

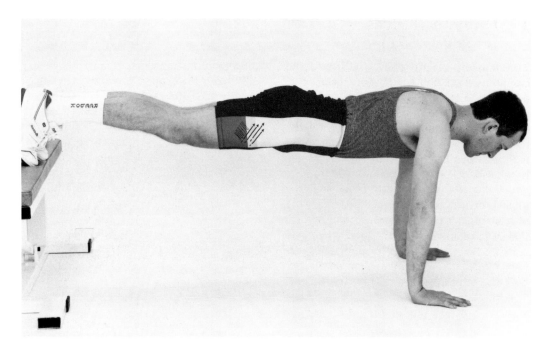

Fig 68 and 69   Bench press-ups.

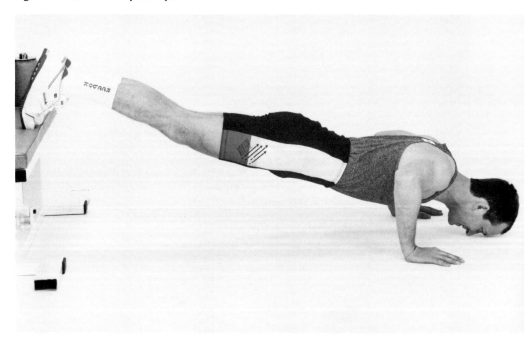

11. Dumb-bell Flyes (*Figs 70 & 71*)

The muscles of the chest can be further conditioned using this exercise. You will need a pair of dumb-bells and a bench. Lie flat on your bench, making sure that your lower back is firmly pressed into the support. Having your feet on the end of the bench makes this easier for some people. Hold a dumb-bell in each hand, elbows slightly bent, with the weights directly above your chest. Now smoothly lower your arms out to the side as far as possible: at this point your hands should be in the same plane as your shoulders. Hold this position, then raise your arms back to the starting position. Breathe in as you lower the weights, and out as you raise them.

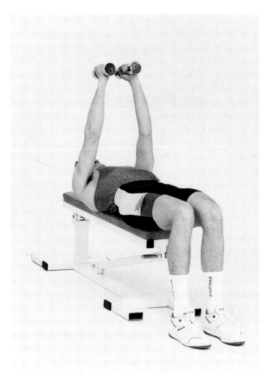

Figs 70 and 71   Dumb-bell flyes.

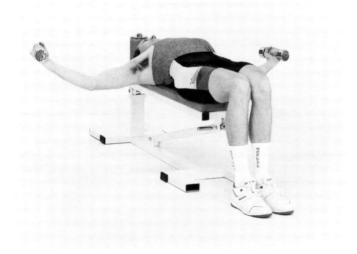

12. Shoulder Press (*Figs 72 & 73*)

This exercise is a great conditioner for the muscles of the shoulders and upper back, as well as the backs of the upper arms. You will need a barbell and a bench or strong chair. Sit tall on your bench with the barbell resting comfortably across your shoulders/upper back. Hold the barbell with a wide grip, elbows under the bar. From this position, press the bar up above your head to arm's length, and then lower it under control until it touches your shoulders again, then repeat. Breathe in as you raise the bar, and out as you lower it. Avoid the temptation to arch your back as you press the bar overhead.

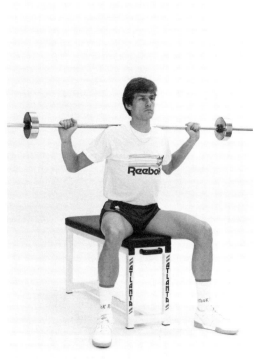
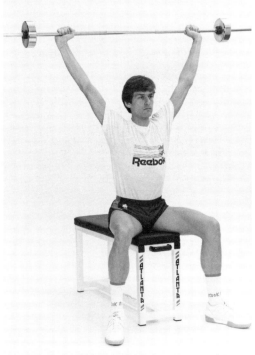

Figs 72 and 73   Shoulder press.

13. Chair Dips
(*Figs 74 & 75*)

In the absence of specialised equipment, you can condition the muscles of the shoulders, upper back and back of the arms using this exercise. You will need a strong chair. Assume the starting position as illustrated. from this position, lower your bottom to the floor by bending at your elbows. Just as your bottom touches the floor, hold this position, then straighten your arms to come back to your starting position, and repeat. Breathe in as you lower to the floor, and out as you return to your starting position. This exercise can be made easier by having your legs bent.

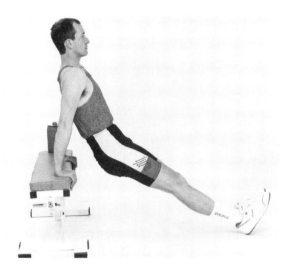

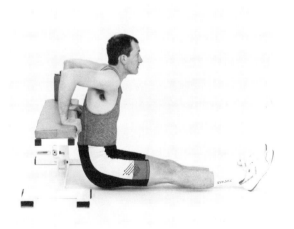

Figs 74 and 75   Chair dips.

14. Lateral Raises (*Fig 76*)

To isolate the muscles of the shoulder, this exercise is very effective. You will need a pair of dumb-bells. Stand tall with your feet about hip-width apart, holding a dumb-bell in each hand, with your elbows slightly bent. From this position, raise the dumb-bells out to the side, taking them to a position where they are approximately in line with your head. Hold this position momentarily, then slowly lower the weights under control to the starting position, and repeat. Breathe in as you raise your arms, and out as you lower them. Be careful in this exercise to keep your trunk stable, avoiding the temptation to throw the dumb-bells upwards.

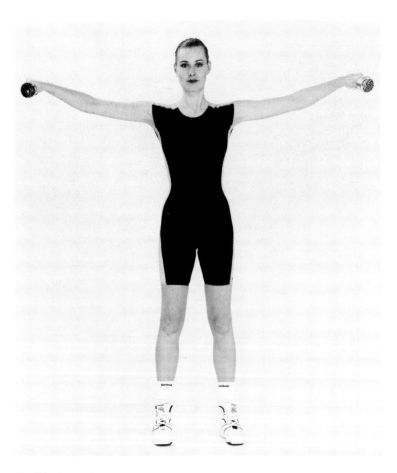

Fig 76   Lateral raises.

15. Upright Rowing (*Figs 77 & 78*)

This is a popular exercise for conditioning the muscles of the upper back and shoulders, as well as those at the front of the upper arms. You will need a barbell. Stand tall, knees slightly bent, with the barbell held with an overgrasp so that your hands are approximately six inches apart. Raise the barbell, keeping it close to the body and keeping your elbows high, so that it ends up in a position opposite your neck. Hold this position for a moment, then slowly lower the barbell back to the starting position, and repeat. Breathe in as you raise the bar, and out as you lower it.

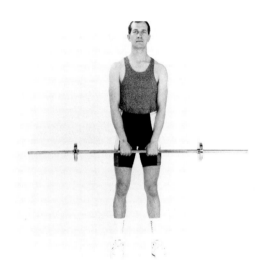 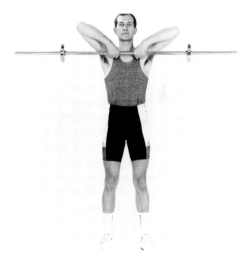

Figs 77 and 78   Upright rowing.

16. Arm Curls
(*Figs 79 & 80*)

This is the basic exercise for conditioning the muscles at the front of the upper arm. It is commonly performed with a barbell, although a pair of dumb-bells can also be used. Stand tall, knees slightly bent, with your feet shoulder-width apart. Hold the barbell with an undergrasp, so that your grip is just wider than your body width. From this position, and keeping your elbows close to your sides, curl the bar up towards your chest, hold your uppermost position for a moment, then slowly lower the bar, under control, back to the starting position. Breathe in as you raise the bar, and out as you lower it.

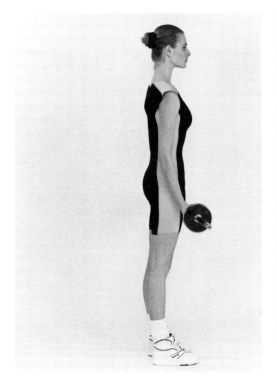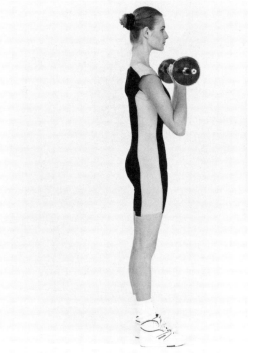

Figs 79 and 80   Arm curls.

STRENGTH PROGRAMMES

The muscular endurance programmes given here can also be used to develop muscular strength. They differ, however, in that heavier resistances are used, only six repetitions of an exercise are required, and instead of moving quickly from exercise to exercise, you repeat the same exercise for the same muscle group after a short recovery phase of approximately 90 seconds. Again, initially through trial and error, choose an exercise position/weight such that you can only just manage six repetitions of the exercise. Rest, and repeat the sequence four times. This is known as 'four sets of six'.

Such programmes are demanding, and also time consuming. If time is of the essence, and you do not mind sacrificing rapid strength gains for average gains, then perform each exercise eight times, moving swiftly on to the next exercise as in the endurance circuit given in *Fig 35*.

It is wise to carry out a general endurance programme for several weeks before beginning a strength programme.

As ever, warm up and warm down thoroughly.

7 Exercise for Improving Flexibility

To improve your range of movement is a relatively simple task, which invariably requires little or no equipment. Essentially all that you need to do is to take your limbs and their associated muscles and joints into a position they have not been in for a while, and hold that position. However, the position that you aim to achieve should be one which is anatomically possible, otherwise injury will be the result. Certain joints and muscles can move safely through some ranges of movement only. These ranges of movement also differ from individual to individual. The dramatic range of movement and general joint mobility associated with classical dancers, for example, is as much inherited as brought about through training. This point is worth bearing in mind in any flexibility programme. You should aim to improve your individual range of movement by following the exercises in Figs 82–91 and the general developmental stretching programme in Fig 81 below, and not worry whether you can do the splits or not.

Before you begin any flexibility programme, you should always make sure that you are warm, since muscles and joint structures in general respond best to any stretching exercise more readily and more effectively once you

---

SAMPLE GENERAL DEVELOPMENTAL STRETCHING PROGRAMME
The preparatory stretching which was carried out as part of your warm-up can be your developmental stretch programme. Modify this by simply holding each stretch for longer: approximately 30 seconds, easing further into the stretch position as the sensation of stretch subsides. There is no need to repeat each stretch more than once.

Neck stretch	(Fig 82)
Diagonal neck stretch	(Fig 83)
Upper back stretch	(Fig 84)
Shoulder and side stretch	(Fig 85)
Chest stretch	(Fig 12)
Side stretch	(Fig 14)
Seated trunk twist	(Fig 86)
Seated groin stretch	(Fig 87)
Lying hamstring stretch	(Fig 88)
Standing quadriceps stretch	(Fig 89)
Standing hip and thigh stretch	
Seated hamstring and groin stretch	(Fig 91)

Fig 81

have warmed up thoroughly. This is the reason why it is recommended in this book that you carry out the bulk of your developmental stretching (that which will lead to an increase in your range of movement) towards the end of your exercise session.

Once you are warm, you should carry out any stretching exercises, such as those given here, paying full attention to the instructions. Position yourself carefully and note that the sensation of stretch that you are feeling once in the appropriate position is indeed the sensation which the instructions indicate that you should be registering. If it is not, it is likely that you are doing something wrong. If all is well, move as far forward into any given stretch as is possible and hold that position, breathing easily throughout the movement. As much as possible, try and relax the rest of the body once in the stretch position. After a few seconds, you may find it possible to move further into the exercise position. If this is the case, do so, and hold your new position. As with all the exercises given in this book, do not try and force your body into any situation, rather ease it carefully and steadily into the exercise. Above all, with stretches do not bounce or fling limbs into a position since this invariably leads to injury.

Whilst there are several methods of stretching to improve flexibility, this method of easing into a position and holding it is one of the simplest and most efficient and carries with it a negligible injury risk if all instructions and guidelines are followed. For preparatory stretching as part of a warm-up phase, any of the stretching exercises can be used in sequence, with each stretch only needing to be held for approximately 6–10 seconds. Developmental stretches aimed at increasing range of movement need to be held a little longer, approximately 20–30 seconds. In each stretching session, do always try and move as far into the exercise positions as possible, since this will ensure progressive improvement.

If you always include some form of comprehensive stretching routine at the end of each exercise session, there is actually no need to add any specific flexibility sessions to your exercise schedule: the careful structuring of each workout so that it incorporates a warm-up and warm-down phase means that flexibility work is incorporated automatically. If you wish to see more rapid increases in range of movement, you can always add extra flexibility programmes to your exercise routine, yet bear in mind that you will have to warm up thoroughly before stretching.

Flexibility exercises may also be used to alleviate muscle soreness associated with strenuous physical activity. Once again, warm up the muscles and joints thoroughly, perhaps even with a hot bath or sauna to begin with, then do the warm-up exercises given earlier, then stretch, easing carefully into the exercise positions and holding them for as long as is comfortable, and keep the affected limbs warm.

As with earlier exercises, you will find instructions for each exercise asking you to sit or stand tall with good posture. Once again, aiming for good posture throughout these exercises will improve their effectiveness.

1. Neck Stretch (*Fig 82*)

Stand or sit tall with good posture. Keeping your neck long, bring your chin towards your chest, feeling the stretch along the back of your neck. Breathe easily throughout. You can make this exercise more demanding by resting your hands loosely on the top of your head as illustrated. Do not pull your head forward.

2. Diagonal Neck Stretch (*Fig 83*)

Stand or sit tall with good posture. With a long neck (shoulders down away from your ears) turn your head to look along the diagonal, before tilting your head and once again bringing your chin towards your chest. You will feel this stretch along the back of the neck and in the upper back muscles. Breathe easily throughout. You can also make this exercise more demanding by resting your hand loosely on the top of your head.

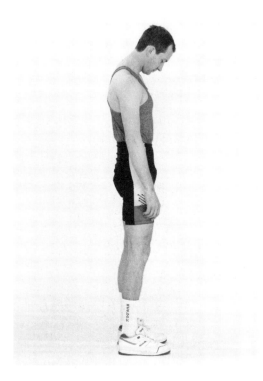

Fig 82   Neck stretch.

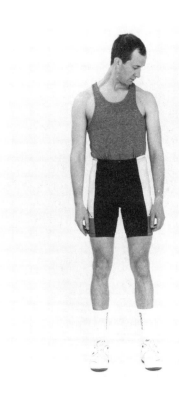

Fig 83   Diagonal neck stretch.

3. Upper Back Stretch (*Fig 84*)

Stand tall with good posture, but with your knees slightly bent and your pelvis tucked under. Interlock your fingers and push your hands away from your chest, looking down and curving your back at the same time. You will feel the stretch between your shoulder blades and along the length of your back. Breathe easily throughout.

4. Shoulder and Side Stretch (*Fig 85*)

Stand tall with good posture, spine long and shoulders down away from your ears. Lift both arms above your head then place your right hand behind the elbow of your left arm and ease your left upper arm behind your head. You will feel the stretch around the shoulder and along the side of your trunk. Repeat on the other side, breathing easily throughout.

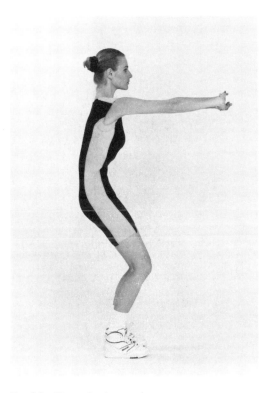

Fig 84   Upper back stretch.

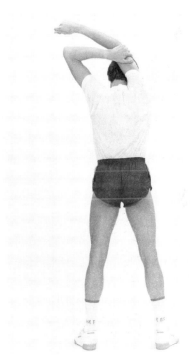

Fig 85   Shoulder and side stretch.

5. Seated Trunk Twist (*Fig 86*)

Sit upright on the floor with your legs stretched out in front of you. Bend the right leg and place your right foot on the outside of the left knee. Twist round so that your shoulders are facing sideways, making sure that your shoulders are still down away from your ears. Use your arms to help you twist round if this helps. Repeat on the other side, breathing easily throughout.

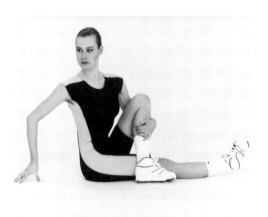

Fig 86   Seated trunk twist.

6. Seated Groin Stretch (*Fig 87*)

Sit tall on the floor with good posture. Bend your knees so that the soles of your feet are together and your knees are out to the side, as close to the floor as possible. Keeping a long spine and your shoulders down away from your ears, relax as much as possible so that your knees fall even closer towards the floor. You will feel the stretch along the inside of the thigh and groin. Use your hands to keep your spine upright, or rest them loosely on your calves. Breathe easily throughout.

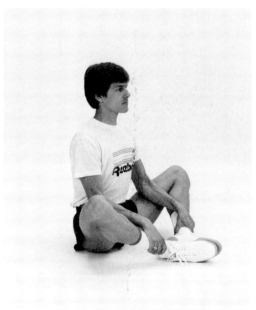

Fig 87   Seated groin stretch.

7. Lying Hamstring Stretch (*Fig 88*)

Lie flat on the floor with your knees bent at approximately 90 degrees. Raise your left leg, grasping it loosely behind the thigh with both hands. Try and straighten this leg and bring it as far as possible towards your chest, still keeping it straight. You will feel the stretch along the back of the outstretched leg. Keep your back and hips pressed against the floor at all times. Repeat on the other side, breathing easily throughout.

8. Standing Quadriceps Stretch (*Fig 89*)

Stand tall with good posture. Hold on to the back of a chair for support and reach behind you with your right arm to loosely grasp your right foot. Gently ease your foot towards your buttocks, whilst still keeping your spine long and your pelvis tucked under and facing forward. You will feel the stretch down the front of the right thigh. Repeat on the other side, breathing easily throughout.

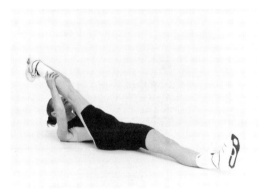

Fig 88   Lying hamstring stretch.

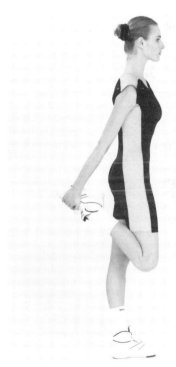

Fig 89   Standing quadriceps stretch.

99

9. Calf Stretches (*Fig 90*)

Stand tall with one leg in front of the other, hands flat against a wall at about shoulder height. Ease your back leg further away from the wall, keeping it straight and press the heel firmly into the floor. Your hips should still be facing forward. Once your leg is far enough away from the wall you will feel the stretch in the calf. Repeat on the other side, breathing easily throughout.

You can stretch the calf lower down by positioning yourself as before, but instead of keeping a straight back leg, bend the knee of this leg slightly, still keeping the heel pressed into the floor. You will feel the stretch more towards the bottom of the calf. Repeat on the other side, breathing easily throughout.

10. Seated Hamstring and Groin Stretch (*Fig 91*)

Sit tall with both legs stretched out in front of you. Bend your right leg to place your right foot against the inside of your left thigh, keeping the right knee close to the floor. Hinge forward from the hips, keeping the back long and reach towards the foot of the straight leg. Hold your furthermost position, feeling the stretch along the back of your outstretched leg and around your groin. Repeat on the other side, breathing easily throughout.

Vary this exercise by allowing your back to round completely, rather than keeping it straight. You will feel more stretch along the back of the straight leg.

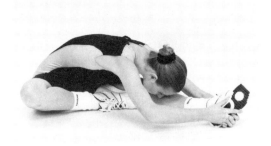

Fig 91   Seated hamstring and groin stretch.

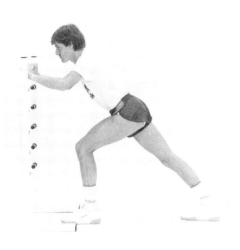

Fig 90   Calf stretches.

8 Your Home Gym

Having read this far, your exercise programme structure, and any equipment you may need in order to carry out your chosen activities, should now be clear. To further illustrate how different people may put together different home exercise programmes according to their fitness goals, likes, dislikes, space and financial restraints, the following profiles of typical home exercisers have been put together. Reading through them all will clearly illustrate that home exercise offers something for everyone.

Andrew, aged 18. A keen runner and rugby player. Wishes to develop strength and flexibility at home. He doesn't have much space and will have to exercise in his bedroom. His finances are also limited.

Since Andrew is already running regularly, and participating in team sports, he is reasonably aerobically fit. To develop strength, he needs to do some form of heavy resistance training, whilst for flexibility, all he really needs to do is follow a developmental stretching programme (*Fig 81*). His best option for general strength training is to purchase a barbell kit. This need not be too heavy to begin with, since he can always purchase extra weight discs as his strength improves, so his initial outlay will be relatively minimal. He can move some of his bedroom furniture to one side to make the space for his exercises. Weight discs and bars can also be stacked under the bed when not in use. An old piece of carpet or non-slip matting will protect the floor surface where he is exercising, and the wardrobe mirror allows him to observe and correct his exercise technique where necessary.

Items purchased: average barbell kit.
Initial outlay: approximately £100.

Carolyn, aged 24. Used to be very active until she moved to her new job. Swims occasionally and does not have much money at present, nor a great deal of space. Has been jogging a couple of times and quite enjoys it. Would basically like to keep fit and trim.

Occasional swimming is not going to keep Carolyn fit. The swimming needs to be more regular, or needs to be combined with some other aerobic activity, in this instance the obvious choice is jogging. If Carolyn aims to jog or swim three times a week, aerobic fitness will be well catered for, as to a certain extent will overall muscular endurance. Extra endurance work can come from the purchase of some wrist/ankle weights in order to carry out a general muscular endurance circuit.

Items purchased: wrist/ankle weights
Initial outlay: approximately £15.

Kate, 28. Has become increasingly inactive as she has pursued her career and has put on quite a bit of weight. Has some money to spend on exercise equipment, but not a great deal of space. Would not enjoy jogging or swimming, but doesn't mind cycling.

Kate's main aim is to improve aerobic fitness and body composition. Essentially this requires increases in energy expenditure through aerobic exercise, and she would also do well to look at her diet. Kate would be well advised to follow a walking programme as well as purchasing an exercise cycle. The walking could be done in her lunch time, with the cycling programme being followed in the evening. The purchase of some wrist/ankle weights will also allow her to follow a general muscular endurance programme.

Items purchased: exercise cycle (£250); wrist/ankle weights (£15).
Initial outlay: approximately £265.

Diana, aged 30. Having two small children, Diana finds herself stuck indoors for a considerable part of the day. Diana and her husband have a spare room in their house and some money, though not a great deal, to spend on exercise equipment. Basically, Diana would just like to 'get fit'.

Once again, the obvious choice for Diana is an exercise cycle and some wrist/ankle weights in order to follow a general muscular endurance programme. The purchase of a fully adjustable exercise cycle also means that her husband can use it, as can the children when they grow a little more. Diana would probably find that it's a good idea to buy a dumb-bell kit for her husband so that he can carry out a comprehensive muscular endurance programme at the same time as she does hers. The spare room makes an ideal venue for her and her husband's exercise programme.

Items purchased: exercise cycle (£250); wrist/ankle weights (£15); dumb-bell kit (£50).
Initial outlay: approximately £315.

Derek, 28 and Heather, 26. Derek and Heather have been married for two years and met through their mutual interest of body-building. They have a large flat but not much money to spend on equipment. Both of them enjoy jogging.

Obviously, both Derek and Heather are enthusiasts. They will be able to train together in their spare room, but will need a substantial amount of equipment, including a bench, stands, barbells and dumb-bells. Scanning the local newspaper ads should enable them to find second-hand equipment relatively cheaply. Jogging will complement their strength and endurance training, as will flexibility work.

Items purchased: bench plus stands (£100); large quantity of weight discs, plus barbells and dumb-bells (£200).
Initial outlay: approximately £300.

Joe, 52 and Doris 56. Both Joe and Doris know that they should exercise more, but they don't. They have plenty of space in their house now that the children have left. Doris enjoys swimming and Joe enjoys walking. Neither of them would like to run, although they both don't mind cycling or rowing. They are financially secure.

There are many options for Joe and Doris. The purchase of an exercise cycle or rowing machine would give them a wider choice of aerobic activities to mix and match in the week and, in so doing, they would not really have to do much additional exercise apart from some flexibility work, since swimming and rowing condition all the major muscle groups of the body.

Items purchased: exercise cycle (£250); rowing ergometer (£600).
Initial outlay: £250 or £850.

Jon, 32. A very keen runner, Jon lives alone in a large flat and has plenty of money. His work means that he finds it increasingly difficult to go out running during the day and he hates running in the evening when it's dark. He would like to improve his running performance and is keen to look at the intensity of his running and train accordingly.

The obvious answer here is a treadmill to run on, plus a heart-rate monitor to gauge with some accuracy the intensity of his running sessions. A small dumb-bell kit will also enable Jon to keep his upper body well conditioned, too.

Items purchased: motorised treadmill (approximately £3,000); heart-rate monitor (£75); small dumb-bell kit (£50).
Initial outlay: £3,125.

The Robinson Family, father 45, mother 40, son 15, daughter 18. Affluent is how you would describe the Robinsons. They have been considering transforming one of their spare rooms into a gym for some time, and have even mirrored one of the walls enabling mother and daughter in the meantime to exercise to an aerobic video. Father and son both run regularly, but would like to do more weight training.

The choice here is obviously a good quality multi-gym, coupled with an exercise bike, and possibly a dumb-bell kit for exercise variety. Each member of the family can use all the equipment, making it a good investment.

Items purchased: good quality multi-gym (£4,000); exercise cycle (£250); dumb-bell kit (£50).
Initial outlay: £4,300.

Obviously, the above are just examples, yet hopefully they serve to show the flexibility of exercising at home.

OTHER CONSIDERATIONS

Apart from space, you should also try and make sure that your exercise environment is a safe and healthy one to work-out in. Exercise surfaces should be non-slip and the room should be airy and well ventilated. Generally speaking, floors do not need strengthening, although if you are purchasing a particularly large multi-gym to be placed in the attic, you may like to check the weight of the equipment with the manufacturer, then consult your builder. If you purchase any items of wall-mounted equipment, check, too that your walls are suitable for the equipment to be attached to. Again, question the manufacturer about the fixing requirements of the equipment.

9 Lifelong Exercise Programming

The most difficult part of any exercise programme for the sedentary individual is the process of getting started. Initial enthusiasm can soon wane, and studies have indicated that the first three to four weeks are crucial. Exercise regularly in this first month, and you're well on the way to exercising for ever. Naturally, as has been stressed throughout this text, you must choose exercise activities which you actually enjoy and which are going to produce the results you are looking for, if you are to exercise for the rest of your life. And exercise need never become boring if you remind yourself that there are many exercise options open to you, and you can always mix and match activities in order to keep motivated.

As an example of this, imagine you have not exercised for several years, in fact, since you left school. You are not particularly keen on any specific exercise activity, perhaps because you have never tried certain activities, or because you didn't like the competitive element of sport which was part and parcel of physical education at school. You would, however, like to do something about your shape, and would like to feel fitter and have more energy.

Your first task is a fitness assessment (Chapter 2). You should then choose an aerobic activity from Chapter 5: any one will do. Let's imagine you choose walking, because it's the easiest to do, and you can fit the programme into a lunch hour, or evening. You should also choose a muscular endurance programme from Chapter 6 and a developmental stretch programme from Chapter 7. Your initial outlay on equipment is minimal, but you're probably wondering how you are going to fit all these exercise activities into a normal working day.

To begin with, notice that for best results from all exercise activities it is recommended that you exercise every other day. This could mean that you do your aerobic programme, your muscular endurance programme and your stretching programme all at the same time, on the same day, in one go. This will take less than 30 minutes when you begin the programme, although as you get fitter, it will take longer, as you need to spend more time exercising to see further improvement. However, you can also fit all your exercise into one day by incorporating two exercise sessions: one for the aerobic programme, carried out, perhaps, at lunch time, and the second combining your endurance and stretching work to be done in the evening. Alternatively, you could do your aerobic programme on one day, and your endurance and flexibility programmes on the next day. In this way, although you are exercising every day, each day's session is different.

After three months, you will be reasonably fit: repeat your fitness assessment to prove it to yourself. You may have got bored with your walking programme (did you vary the routes enough?) and fed up with the endurance and flexibility programmes. If this is the case, change everything. Try a jogging programme, and either change the exercises you are doing in the endurance and flexibility programmes, or give yourself a new challenge in the form of a strength programme. Try this combination out for a few months, see what effect it's having on you, reassess, and then make a fresh activity plan. This time it could be cycling, plus one general endurance session, one strength session and one endurance/ aerobic session per week. There is no reason why you should not mix up your activities to provide variety. Naturally, you need to have some kind of plan so that you are achieving a measure of systematic conditioning. Logging your activities will enable you to see whether you are neglecting a certain type of activity for any length of time.

Just as you may mix up your endurance/ strength activities and programmes, so you can mix up your aerobic activities. If you get bored running every other day, try cycling, or rowing, or something else from the aerobic list on one of your running days. Obviously, if you are aiming to enter running races, this is not such a good idea, since you will not be conditioning your body to the demands of running, but if general fitness is your aim, swapping an activity, and carrying it out at the same relative intensity and duration adds for variety and can alleviate boredom. In other words, the important aspect as far as life-long training is concerned is variety. Do not think you always have to exercise in the same way. Vary the activities, the exercises, the programmes. Be flexible. As long as you follow the exercise and training guidelines given in this book, you will achieve results.

Some people find other ways of keeping motivated. Challenging oneself certainly works for many people. So if you are a runner, you may like to enter fun runs and races, and log your best times for certain distances. You can also do this on other aerobic equipment, looking for personal bests for certain distances on a cycle or rowing machine. Do not try and perform a personal best on every exercise session, however, since

working flat out like this introduces a high injury risk: once every few weeks is probably about right.

Other regular exercisers keep exercising with the help of a training or exercise partner. Many exercises and activities lend themselves to being done in pairs or in a group, walking and running being obvious examples. This introduces a social aspect to the exercise programme which many people need and enjoy. Arranging to meet someone at a certain time to exercise with them also makes it that much harder to break your commitment to that exercise session.

INTERRUPTIONS TO TRAINING

Occasionally you will find that events occuring over a few days will interrupt your training programme. Holidays and illness are obvious examples. A holiday is the easiest to deal with and viewed in a different light, can actually improve your training and fitness level. Use the holiday environment to try out different exercise activities or programmes. So, for instance, experiment with running on the beach (very demanding if done on soft sand), walking up hills, swimming, and cycling to beauty spots/ historic ruins (most holiday resorts have cycle hire facilities). With a little thought, any holiday can be made more active, and the different exercise environment makes the activity all the more enjoyable and interesting.

You can also structure a simple endurance/ aerobic circuit of exercises from those given in the warm-up section (Chapter 4) and from those given in Chapter 6, which can easily be carried out in your hotel room, as indicated in *Fig 92*.

Illness or injury poses more of a problem than going away on holiday. If you are laid up for up to a week, you should be able to ease

105

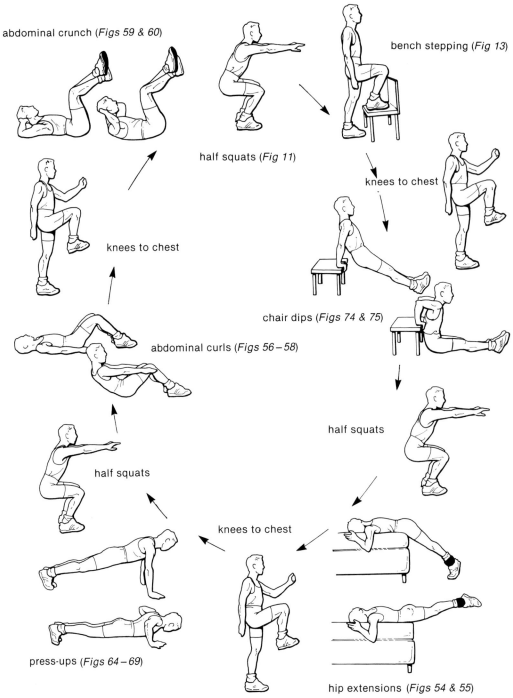

abdominal crunch (*Figs 59 & 60*)

bench stepping (*Fig 13*)

half squats (*Fig 11*)

knees to chest

knees to chest

chair dips (*Figs 74 & 75*)

abdominal curls (*Figs 56 – 58*)

half squats

half squats

knees to chest

press-ups (*Figs 64 – 69*)

hip extensions (*Figs 54 & 55*)

Fig 92   Hotel exercise circuit.

Hotel exercise circuit

WARM-UP, PLUS PREPARATORY STRETCHING

30 seconds of half squats	*(Fig 11)*
Bench stepping (use a chair) (15 repeats)	*(Fig 13)*
30 seconds of knees to chest	
Chair dips (15 repeats)	*(Figs 74 & 75)*
30 seconds of half squats	
Hip extensions	*(Figs 55 & 56)*
30 seconds of knees to chest	
Press-ups (15 repeats)	*(Figs 64 – 68)*
30 seconds of half squats	
Abdominal curls	*(Figs 57 – 59)*
30 seconds of knees to chest	
Abdominal crunch	*(Figs 60 & 61)*

Repeat the circuit up to 3 times in succession, according to fitness.
Warm down thoroughly.
Perform every other day.

Fig 92

yourself back into your exercise programme relatively quickly. Do not go back to what you were doing prior to your illness, rather, work at a lower intensity for a couple of sessions before going back to your original programme.

The longer you are away from exercise, the more gradual must be your return. After several weeks of relative inactivity, it is worthwhile reassessing your fitness level and going to a level in your activity programme which is suitable. Do not rush back into physical activity after a lay off – you are likely to injure yourself and lose even more weeks of training.

Useful Addresses

EQUIPMENT SUPPLIERS

Most major sports stores will be able to supply most of the equipment listed and mentioned in the text. If you have any difficulty, the following manufacturers/distributors should be able to help.

Fitness Testing Equipment

Command Electronics (Heart-rate monitors)
189/191 London Road
Mitcham
Surrey
CR4 2JB

BodyCare Products Ltd
57 Fieldgate Lane
Kenilworth
Warwickshire
CV8 1BT

Health Promotion (UK) Ltd
23 Chilworth Mews
London
W2 3RG

The National Coaching Foundation
4 College Close
Beckett Park
Leeds
West Yorkshire
LS6 3QH

SLM
Unit 2
New Inn Bridge Estate
998 Foleshill Road
Coventry
West Midlands
CV6 6NE

Home Exercise Equipment (Weights, benches, cycles, treadmills, etc.)

Atlanta Sports Industries
Atlanta House
Denby Way
Euroway Estate
Hellaby, Maltby
Rotherham
South Yorkshire
S66 8QN

Bolton Stirland International
Boland House
Nottingham South Industrial Estate
Ruddington Lane
Wilford
Nottingham
Nottinghamshire
NG11 7EP

Concept II Rowing Ergometer
Concept II
151 – 153 Nottingham Road
Old Basford
Nottingham
Nottinghamshire
NG6 0FU

Kettler (GB) Ltd
Kettler House
Merse Road
North Moons Moat
Redditch
Worcestershire
B98 9HL

Kynex Ltd
Drummond House
94 Broad Street
Birmingham
West Midlands
B15 1AU

Life Fitness
Queen Adelaide
Ely
Cambridgeshire
CB7 4UB

Polaris (Sports Equipment) Ltd
Norman House
Heritage Gate
Derby
Derbyshire
DE1 1NU

Power Sport International
Queens Road
Bridgend Industrial Estate
Bridgend
Mid Glamorgan
CF31 3UE

J. Schnell (UK) Ltd
250 Durnsford Road
London
SW19 6DS

York Barbell (UK) Ltd
Unit 4/5 High March
Daventry
Northamptonshire
NN11 4NF

Index